The Alzheimer's Disease Mastery Bible: Your Blueprint For Complete Alzheimer's Disease Management

Dr. Ankita Kashyap and Prof. Krishna N. Sharma

Published by Virtued Press, 2023.

While every precaution has been taken in the preparation of this book, the publisher assumes no responsibility for errors or omissions, or for damages resulting from the use of the information contained herein.

THE ALZHEIMER'S DISEASE MASTERY BIBLE: YOUR BLUEPRINT FOR COMPLETE ALZHEIMER'S DISEASE MANAGEMENT

First edition. November 20, 2023.

Copyright © 2023 Dr. Ankita Kashyap and Prof. Krishna N. Sharma.

ISBN: 979-8223883500

Written by Dr. Ankita Kashyap and Prof. Krishna N. Sharma.

Table of Contents

DISCLAIMER

The information provided in this book is intended for general informational purposes only. The content is not meant to substitute professional medical advice, diagnosis, or treatment. Always consult with a qualified healthcare provider before making any changes to your diabetes management plan or healthcare regimen.

While every effort has been made to ensure the accuracy and completeness of the information presented, the author and publisher do not assume any responsibility for errors, omissions, or potential misinterpretations of the content. Individual responses to diabetes management strategies may vary, and what works for one person might not be suitable for another.

The book does not endorse any specific medical treatments, products, or services. Readers are encouraged to seek guidance from their healthcare providers to determine the most appropriate approaches for their unique medical conditions and needs.

Any external links or resources provided in the book are for convenience and informational purposes only. The author and publisher do not have control over the content or availability of these external sources and do not endorse or guarantee the accuracy of such information.

Readers are advised to exercise caution and use their judgment when applying the information provided in this book to their own situations. The author and publisher disclaim any liability for any direct, indirect, consequential, or other damages arising from the use of this book and its content.

By reading and using this book, readers acknowledge and accept the limitations and inherent risks associated with implementing the strategies, recommendations, and information contained herein. It is always recommended to consult a qualified healthcare professional for personalized medical advice and care.

Introduction

A remarkable book named "The Alzheimer's Disease Mastery Bible: Your Blueprint for Complete Alzheimer's Disease Management" once existed in a world full of inquisitive minds and enthusiastic souls. It was a magnificent book that was so expertly made that it seemed to pulse with the ability to change people's lives. Written by none other than the extraordinary Dr. Ankita Kashyap, this literary gem offered hope to people enduring the perilous path of Alzheimer's disease.

Dr. Kashyap became a beacon of wisdom in a world full of confusing terminology and medical jargon. He was a skilled writer with an aptitude for understanding the subtleties of this ailment that could change people's minds. Equipped with her extensive medical knowledge and her steadfast dedication to advocating for holistic healthcare, she set out on a mission to provide knowledge, comprehension, and a touch of humour to individuals suffering from Alzheimer's Disease.

I was taken to a world where compassion and science coexisted together as I read this captivating book; words painted vivid pictures on the canvas of comprehension. Like a kind sorcerer, Dr. Kashyap pulled us into her world and asked us to enjoy the adventure that lay ahead. I could feel the wide breadth of her research with each page flip, the many hours she devoted to reading reliable medical publications and scientific studies. It was evidence of her steadfast devotion to accuracy and truth, as well as her desire to discovering the mysteries of this odd illness.

However, this book's capacity to go beyond the confines of conventional medical literature was what really set it apart. Dr. Kashyap created an educational and entertaining knowledge-based tapestry with her skillful storytelling. Her soft voice sounded like it was whispering in my ear as I read, guiding me through this journey's turns and turns. She interpreted the intricate medical ideas with ease and precision, balancing them with compassion and comprehension. She added a dash of clarity to every statement so that even the most complex concepts were understandable to all.

The author's words danced over the pages, conjuring up vibrant images of resiliency, optimism, and limitless possibilities. They dipped in and out of the lives of those suffering from Alzheimer's, accepting their particular worries and anxieties. Dr. Kashyap provided a thorough and well-rounded approach to managing diseases by skillfully combining medical and holistic health viewpoints through her rigorous organisation. With each chapter, the author skillfully addressed the unique requirements of individuals impacted by Alzheimer's Disease, creating a symphony of insights.

However, this wasn't your typical self-help book. Because every person's experience with Alzheimer's disease is as different as a snowflake, Dr. Kashyap developed individualised programmes and self-help methods that let readers adjust their treatment approaches to suit their particular situation. It demonstrated her steadfast faith in the capabilities of flexibility and relevance, which reverberated across this masterpiece's pages. She realised that there was no one-size-fits-all approach to managing Alzheimer's disease; rather, it required a patchwork of individualised care, nurturing, and development.

Dr. Ankita Kashyap has established a safe haven for anyone navigating the unpredictable path of Alzheimer's disease in her book, "The Alzheimer's Disease Mastery Bible: Your Blueprint for Complete Alzheimer's Disease Management." She had created a lighthouse of comprehension, optimism, and tremendous healing. A feeling of wonder pervaded the air as I closed the book because I knew that behind its pages lied the ability to change, heal, and release.

I so extend an invitation to you, my reader, to enter this realm of wisdom and wonder. Grab hold of this amazing book, allow its words to soothe your spirit, and set off on a trip that will change your perspective on Alzheimer's disease forever. Accept the magic that these pages hold, for they contain your guide to managing Alzheimer's disease in its entirety. Come with me on this incredible journey, since information alone will enable us to successfully negotiate the winding routes of this mysterious illness. Together, let's solve the puzzles, reveal the secrets, and realise the countless opportunities that lie ahead.

Welcome, dear reader, to a world where every single one of us has the capacity to transform, where optimism and science coexist, and where compassion and medicine meet. The one and only Dr. Ankita Kashyap welcomes you to "The Alzheimer's Disease Mastery Bible: Your Blueprint for Complete Alzheimer's Disease Management."

Chapter 1: Understanding Alzheimer's Disease

The Biology of Alzheimer's Disease

Amyloid plaques are frequently the first thing that spring to mind when we think of Alzheimer's disease. The aberrant protein known as amyloid-beta builds up in the brain to produce these plaques. Amyloid-beta is a sticky material that aggregates to produce insoluble plaques that impede brain cell activity.

An imbalance between the brain's production and clearance of amyloid-beta leads to the accumulation of amyloid plaques. Normally, a sensitive system produces and eliminates amyloid-beta. But in Alzheimer's disease patients, this clearing procedure gets overburdened and ineffective. Consequently, amyloid-beta builds up and creates plaques, impairing the brain's regular operation.

Although amyloid plaques are a characteristic feature of Alzheimer's disease, other factors also play a role in the disease's development. The tau protein, which creates twisted tangles inside brain cells, is another important component in the illness process. Tau protein is crucial for preserving the stability and form of nerve cells, but Alzheimer's disease causes it to undergo aberrant modification and cluster together, which results in the buildup of insoluble tangles.

These tau tangles interfere with neurons' ability to communicate with one another and eventually lead to the death of the neurons. In patients with Alzheimer's disease, the amount of tau tangles is tightly correlated with the rate at which cognitive impairment advances. Actually, compared to amyloid plaque load, tau pathology may be a more accurate indicator of cognitive impairment, according to new studies.

Neuroinflammation is a major factor in the onset and progression of Alzheimer's disease, in addition to the buildup of tau tangles and amyloid plaques. A physiological reaction to damage or infection in the brain, neuroinflammation is characterised by immune cell activation and the release of inflammatory chemicals.

Chronic neuroinflammation in Alzheimer's disease is brought on by the protracted buildup of tau tangles and amyloid plaques. Neuronal injury is worsened by the production of inflammatory chemicals by activated immune cells in the brain, such as astrocytes and microglia.

A number of proposals have been put out, but the precise pathways tying neuroinflammation, tau tangles, and amyloid plaques in Alzheimer's disease are still unclear. According to one theory, tau disease results from immune cells being activated by amyloid-beta, which then causes the production of inflammatory mediators. According to a different view, tau tangles themselves might cause neuroinflammation, which would then continue the vicious cycle of inflammation and neuronal destruction.

It is evident that the interaction of tau tangles, neuroinflammation, and amyloid plaques leads to the neurodegenerative processes seen in Alzheimer's disease, regardless of the precise causal links. Comprehending these pathways is essential for the creation of tailored treatments that can successfully halt the advancement of the illness.

Drug development efforts are under progress to create medications that specifically target tau and amyloid-beta proteins and encourage their removal from the brain. Furthermore, preclinical research has demonstrated the potential of anti-inflammatory drugs to reduce neuroinflammation. For the millions of people suffering from this terrible illness, these promising treatments may be the key to delaying or perhaps stopping the disease's course.

In summary, the biology of Alzheimer's disease is a complicated network of related mechanisms. The formation and course of the disease are attributed to tau tangles, neuroinflammation, and amyloid plaques, which ultimately result in cognitive decline and functional impairment. It is essential to comprehend the functions of these biological processes in order to create efficient management and treatment plans for Alzheimer's disease. The devastation caused by Alzheimer's disease may be slowed down or perhaps prevented by focusing on these processes, which would ultimately improve the lives of those who have the illness and their loved ones.

Genetic Factors and Risk

Recent developments in the study of genetics have illuminated the intricate relationship between genes and illness risk. Although much remains to be discovered, a number of genes have been shown to increase the likelihood of Alzheimer's disease. The apolipoprotein E (APOE) gene is one such gene.

The APOE gene contributes to the synthesis of apolipoprotein E, a protein that is involved in the brain's lipid and cholesterol metabolism. Research has indicated that this gene has three prevalent variants, or alleles: APOE ε2, APOE ε3, and APOE ε4. There is a distinct risk associated with each of these alleles for Alzheimer's disease.

Compared to people without the APOE ε4 allele, those who carry it have a higher chance of acquiring Alzheimer's disease. Actually, the chance of contracting the condition increases two to three times with one copy of the APOE ε4 allele and ten to fifteen times with two copies. However, it has been discovered that the APOE ε2 allele is linked to a lower risk of Alzheimer's disease.

The age at which Alzheimer's disease first appears is influenced by the APOE ε4 allele, which also raises the disease's likelihood of occurrence. According to studies, those who have this gene typically get the disease sooner in life than people who do not. This information enables early intervention and management of Alzheimer's disease and is crucial in identifying those who may be more vulnerable to the disease.

The presenilin 1 (PSEN1) gene is another one that has attracted a lot of interest in the field of Alzheimer's disease research. Rare types of early-onset familial Alzheimer's disease, which usually manifest before the age of 60, have been linked to mutations in this gene. These mutations significantly affect an individual's vulnerability to disease, and those who carry them have an almost 100% probability of getting Alzheimer's disease.

The presenilin genes, which include PSEN1, produce the presenilin protein, which is a component of a complex that aids in the processing of the amyloid precursor protein (APP). Alzheimer's disease is characterised by the buildup of amyloid-beta plaques, which are caused by mutations in the PSEN1 gene.

Apart from the APOE and PSEN1 genes, there exist multiple other genes that have been found to be associated with the risk of Alzheimer's disease. These include the amyloid precursor protein (APP) gene and the presenilin 2 (PSEN2) gene, which is also linked to early-onset familial Alzheimer's disease.

Comprehending the genetic component of Alzheimer's disease holds significance not just for scientific purposes but also for its use in clinical settings. Genetic testing can assist in identifying those who could be more susceptible to the illness, enabling early intervention and individualised treatment plans. Additionally, knowing the hereditary components of Alzheimer's disease can aid in the creation of tailored treatments meant to halt or delay the illness's progression.

But it's crucial to keep in mind that, when it comes to Alzheimer's disease, heredity is just one component of the picture. Although certain hereditary variables may raise the likelihood of the disease occurring, they do not ensure it will. Diet, exercise, sleep patterns, and stress reduction are examples of lifestyle factors that significantly influence an individual's vulnerability to disease.

In my experience as a health and wellness coach, lifestyle changes have a profoundly positive impact on the management of Alzheimer's disease. Through the implementation of a comprehensive strategy that integrates genetics, lifestyle adjustments, and individualised assistance, people can enhance their cognitive well-being and reduce their likelihood of Alzheimer's disease.

In summary, a person's genetic makeup greatly influences their chance of acquiring Alzheimer's disease. The vulnerability to Alzheimer's disease has been linked to genes like APOE and PSEN1, which influence the age at which the disease manifests as well as the probability of acquiring Alzheimer's disease. Knowing these genetic variables enables tailored management plans and early intervention. But it's important to understand that lifestyle choices can have a big impact on illness vulnerability; genetics is just one piece of the jigsaw. Through a comprehensive strategy that integrates genetics, lifestyle changes, and individualised assistance, people can take charge of their mental well-being and reduce their chance of developing Alzheimer's disease.

Early Signs and Symptoms

A person's cognitive abilities and behaviour may first show mild, subtle alterations as they go through Alzheimer's disease. These alterations could be simply written off as a typical aspect of ageing or linked to weariness or stress. But, it is imperative that you take note of these warning indicators and seek prompt medical attention because early treatment can significantly enhance quality of life and halt the disease's progression.

Memory loss is among the first and most prevalent symptoms of Alzheimer's disease. While occasional forgetfulness is common, chronic memory issues that cause challenges in day-to-day functioning may be cause for concern. People could ask for the same information again, forget significant dates or occasions, or rely largely on notes or reminders to help them remember things. They can also start losing things and find it tough to go back.

Alzheimer's disease can impair a person's capacity to reason and think clearly in addition to causing memory loss. They might struggle to focus, plan their ideas, or come to decisions. Things that were easy and comfortable at first can become difficult and perplexing. They can find it difficult to pay attention in class or follow directions. The independence and day-to-day functioning of an individual might be greatly impacted by these cognitive deficiencies.

Another early indication of Alzheimer's disease is difficulty speaking and interacting with others. People could find it difficult to follow discussions, struggle to find the correct words, or repeat themselves a lot. Additionally, they might have trouble writing or reading, and over time, their spoken or written language might become less intelligible. These shifts in communication abilities are sometimes mistaken for stress or age-related decline.

People may experience behavioural and emotional changes as their Alzheimer's disease worsens. They could lose interest in things they used to appreciate and turn apathetic. They could shy away from people and want to be by themselves. However, some people might experience agitation, anxiety, or irritability. They might go through abrupt mood swings or behave in an unusual way. These adjustments may have an adverse effect on their own health as well as their relationships with family and caregivers.

Moreover, insomnia may be a precursor of Alzheimer's disease. People may suffer from nightmares or vivid dreams, have difficulty falling or staying asleep, or have restless or irregular sleep patterns. Sleep disturbances might worsen cognitive deficits and heighten perplexity and disorientation in general.

Finding an early diagnosis and beginning Alzheimer's disease treatment begins with recognising these warning signs and symptoms. It's critical to realise that these symptoms might differ from person to person and don't always point to Alzheimer's disease. However, it is imperative to seek a comprehensive examination from a healthcare provider if you or a loved one is exhibiting persistent behavioural and cognitive changes that are creating concern and interfering with day-to-day activities.

Prompt diagnosis facilitates timely treatment and aids in future planning for both people and families. It offers the chance to look into the support programmes that are accessible, get caregiver resources, and make wise financial and legal decisions. Early intervention can also support people in participating in activities that enhance their well-being and cognitive health as well as helping them keep their independence for longer.

In conclusion, early diagnosis and intervention for Alzheimer's Disease depend on the ability to recognise the disease's early indications and symptoms. In my capacity as a physician and health and wellness coach, I advise patients and their families to exercise caution and to get checked out if they observe long-lasting behavioural and cognitive abnormalities. We can successfully manage Alzheimer's disease and enhance the quality of life for both patients and their carers by being proactive and obtaining the right support. Recall that information is power, and that by working together, we can defeat Alzheimer's.

Diagnostic Tools and Tests

A thorough medical and cognitive evaluation is often the first step on the path to an Alzheimer's diagnosis. When assessing a patient's memory, cognitive function, and reasoning skills, cognitive evaluations are essential. These evaluations are frequently carried out by neuropsychologists who are skilled in identifying and analysing the cognitive alterations linked to Alzheimer's disease. A battery of standardised tests measuring many components of cognitive function, including memory, language, attention, and problem-solving abilities, are usually used in these evaluations.

Patients may be required to perform tasks like word recall, puzzle solving, or following directions during these evaluations. The outcomes of these evaluations offer insightful information about the patient's cognitive functioning and assist in locating any possible deterioration that might be suggestive of Alzheimer's disease. It is significant to remember that these cognitive tests serve as the cornerstone of the diagnostic procedure, offering a thorough comprehension of the patient's cognitive deficits.

Brain imaging is essential for the diagnosis of Alzheimer's disease in addition to cognitive tests. The two most used imaging methods for diagnosing Alzheimer's disease are computed tomography (CT) scans and magnetic resonance imaging (MRI). With the use of these imaging techniques, medical practitioners can examine the brain in great detail and search for any obvious abnormalities or structural changes. Brain imaging in Alzheimer's disease can show patterns of brain atrophy, especially in the hippocampus and frontal lobes, two regions of the brain important in memory and cognition.

Furthermore, brain function and metabolism can be assessed with positron emission tomography (PET) scans. A radioactive tracer that can bind to beta-amyloid plaques, a defining feature of Alzheimer's disease, is administered during a PET scan. Through the visualisation of beta-amyloid plaque buildup and distribution inside the brain, PET scans offer a more precise assessment of the pathology that underlies Alzheimer's disease. Furthermore, as a decrease in glucose metabolism is frequently seen in people with Alzheimer's disease, PET scans can also be used to evaluate glucose metabolism in the brain.

Although cognitive tests and brain imaging offer insightful information, the discovery of biomarkers has brought about tremendous progress in the study of Alzheimer's disease. Biomarkers are biological signs that can be detected in bodily fluids like blood or CSF. They can offer important hints regarding the onset and course of Alzheimer's disease. The most well-known proteins like tau and beta-amyloid are biomarkers linked to Alzheimer's disease.

Analyzing cerebrospinal fluid (CSF) is one way to quantify these indicators. Through lumbar puncture, medical personnel can get a small sample of cerebrospinal fluid and measure the amounts of tau and beta-amyloid proteins. Increased tau and amyloid-beta protein levels are frequently seen in Alzheimer's patients and can provide compelling evidence for a diagnosis. It's crucial to remember that lumbar punctures have dangers and complications of their own and should only be performed by qualified medical personnel.

Blood tests are a promising new tool for biomarker research. Researchers have been looking into the prospect of finding biomarkers specific to Alzheimer's disease in blood samples since they offer a more accessible and less intrusive diagnostic method. Certain proteins, such tau and amyloid-beta, can be found in blood samples and may be biomarkers for Alzheimer's disease, according to a number of studies. The identification of reliable blood markers for Alzheimer's disease has the potential to completely transform the diagnostic procedure by increasing its effectiveness and accessibility.

A patient's medical history, including any genetic predispositions or risk factors, should be well understood in addition to cognitive evaluations, brain imaging, and biomarker analysis. It is critical to take into account the patient's general health, prescription drugs, and any co-occurring illnesses that could affect cognitive performance. Comprehending the patient's general health and lifestyle is a crucial aspect of the diagnostic procedure, as it facilitates the creation of an all-encompassing treatment strategy.

To sum up, a precise diagnosis is essential for managing Alzheimer's disease effectively. Brain imaging, biomarker analysis, and cognitive tests are commonly included in the diagnostic process. Cognitive tests aid in assessing the patient's cognitive abilities, and brain imaging sheds light on anatomical changes in the brain. Using CSF or blood samples, biomarker analysis provides insight into the onset and course of Alzheimer's disease. Healthcare providers can create individualised management programmes that cater to the specific requirements of each patient and advance holistic health and wellness by integrating various diagnostic tools and tests.

Stages of Alzheimer's Disease

Stage 1: Preclinical Alzheimer's Disease

Alzheimer's disease symptoms might not be immediately noticeable in the early stages. There may be mild alterations in the brain during this preclinical period, but there are no obvious memory issues or cognitive decline. The accumulation of tau tangles and beta-amyloid plaques, the two main brain abnormalities linked to Alzheimer's disease, starts at this point.

Even while people with preclinical Alzheimer's disease might not exhibit any overt symptoms, it's still critical to begin leading a healthy lifestyle and using techniques that promote brain health. This entails having a healthy diet, exercising frequently, and taking part in mentally challenging activities.

I frequently advise my patients to take part in planned activities that can help keep their wits sharp and stimulated, such reading, solving puzzles, picking up a new instrument, or learning a language. By fostering cognitive reserve, these activities can help preserve cognitive function and postpone the development of symptoms.

Stage 2: Mild Cognitive Impairment (MCI) due to Alzheimer's Disease

MCI is a stage at which people start to exhibit subtle cognitive and memory abnormalities that are apparent to both them and everyone around them. Even though these modifications might not have a major effect on day-to-day functioning, they can be concerning since they might point to the early stages of Alzheimer's disease.

It's critical to have a thorough evaluation done at this point in order to rule out other possible explanations and identify the underlying source of the cognitive deterioration. This may entail performing a thorough medical examination, cognitive assessments, and brain imaging.

Upon confirmation of an MCI caused by Alzheimer's disease diagnosis, it is imperative to put procedures in place to support cognitive function and control symptoms. Participating in cognitive rehabilitation programmes, which could include memory drills and cognitive training, may be one way to achieve this. These courses are designed to strengthen cognitive abilities and memory.

It becomes even more crucial to maintain a healthy lifestyle in addition to these measures. A balanced diet, consistent exercise, enough sleep, and stress reduction practises can all help to support the health of the brain overall.

Maintaining a supportive network and participating in social events are also crucial. Feelings of depression and isolation, which are frequent among people with mild cognitive impairment, can be lessened by social activity and maintaining relationships with loved ones.

Stage 3: Mild Alzheimer's Disease

People with Alzheimer's disease eventually reach the mild stage, which is characterised by increasingly pronounced cognitive and functional losses. It may become apparent that there is memory loss, trouble making decisions and solving problems, and difficulty finishing chores that are known to you.

It is critical to put procedures into place at this point to control symptoms and preserve quality of life. Adding structure and procedures to everyday tasks is one useful strategy. Establishing a regular routine and creating a predictable environment can help people with moderate Alzheimer's disease feel less anxious and more grounded.

Using assistive technologies and memory aides can also be helpful. Calendars, to-do lists, reminder applications, and prescription organisers are a few examples of these. These tools can assist people in maintaining organisation and improving the efficiency of their daily work.

In this phase, caregivers are also essential since they offer support and help when needed. A caring approach and transparent communication are crucial while attending to the demands and worries of the person suffering from Alzheimer's disease.

Stage 4: Moderate Alzheimer's Disease

The cognitive and functional impairment in Alzheimer's disease increases during its moderate stage. As memory loss worsens, people may find it difficult to identify familiar persons and locations. Additionally, they could struggle with language, which makes communication difficult.

At this point, making sure everyone is safe takes precedence. It's critical to install safety equipment and eliminate potential threats to create a safe and secure atmosphere at home. Furthermore, caregivers can want extra help with routine tasks like eating, dressing, and bathing.

It might also be advantageous to put communication support tactics into practise. This entails using gestures and facial expressions to help understanding, speaking quietly and clearly, and making use of visual signals. Participating in activities that encourage reflection and fortify ties to cherished memories, such flipping through photo albums or listening to well-known music, can also be beneficial.

Stage 5: Severe Alzheimer's Disease

People with Alzheimer's disease who are in the severe stages of the disease have significant cognitive and functional impairment. They might not be able to recognise loved ones or speak verbally, and they might need complete support with everyday tasks.

At this point, the emphasis switches to comfort and preserving the person's quality of life. This can entail offering tactile, visual, and auditory stimulation—for example, by utilising aromatherapy or relaxing music. It is imperative to guarantee adequate nourishment and hydration, since swallowing challenges could surface during this phase.

Together, medical experts and caregivers provide compassionate care that ensures the patient's physical, emotional, and mental well. Services for hospice and palliative care may be sought to offer further assistance and direction at this point.

In summary, sustaining quality of life and controlling symptoms of Alzheimer's disease require a grasp of the illness's stages. We can assist people with Alzheimer's disease and their carers in navigating this difficult journey by putting into practise the right tactics and interventions at each step.

Risk Factors and Prevention

I have devoted my professional life to advancing holistic healthcare and wellbeing as a physician and health and wellness coach. I serve patients in my office with a team of specialists from different wellness and health sectors, giving them a complete approach to maintaining their health. One of the things I concentrate on when it comes to Alzheimer's disease is identifying the modifiable risk factors and putting preventative measures in place that can assist lower the likelihood of getting the illness.

I will explore the modifiable risk factors for Alzheimer's disease in this subchapter, along with lifestyle modifications and preventative strategies that can be used to lower the risk. While some risk factors, like age and heredity, are unavoidable, there are a number of things that we can control that can significantly affect our brain health and lower our chance of acquiring Alzheimer's disease.

Let's start by discussing one of the most significant controllable risk factors: lifestyle. Our everyday routines and decisions about food, exercise, sleep, stress reduction, and social interaction can all have an effect on the health of our brains. We can lower the risk of Alzheimer's disease and establish a protective environment for our brains by deliberately working to prioritise these areas.

A healthy diet is essential for preserving brain function. According to research, the risk of Alzheimer's disease can be considerably reduced by eating a diet high in fruits, vegetables, whole grains, lean proteins, and healthy fats like those in nuts, olive oil, and oily salmon. These meals include vital nutrients and antioxidants that assist in shielding the brain against inflammation and oxidative stress. Conversely, a diet heavy in processed foods, sugar-filled beverages, and unhealthy fats may make cognitive decline more likely. Thus, the key to preventing Alzheimer's disease is adopting intelligent dietary decisions.

Exercise is a vital component in managing one's lifestyle. Numerous advantages of regular physical activity for brain health have been demonstrated. It improves memory and cognitive function, stimulates the development of new neurons, and boosts blood flow to the brain. Alzheimer's disease risk can be considerably decreased by doing cardiovascular exercise for at least 150 minutes each week, such as jogging, cycling, swimming, or brisk walking. The health of the brain is further improved when aerobic exercises are combined with strength training activities like yoga or weightlifting. Consequently, one of the most important things we can do to lower our risk of Alzheimer's disease is to exercise every day.

Research indicates that poor sleep quality or chronic sleep deprivation can raise the risk of cognitive decline and Alzheimer's disease, despite the fact that sleep is frequently disregarded as a crucial component of brain health. The brain goes through significant processes that detoxify and solidify memories when we sleep. Thus, maintaining brain health and preventing Alzheimer's disease requires receiving enough good sleep—ideally between 7-9 hours per night.

Another essential component of preventing Alzheimer's disease is stress management. Prolonged stress can harm the brain and raise the possibility of cognitive impairment. Using stress-reduction strategies, such as deep breathing exercises, mindfulness meditation, or taking up enjoyable and relaxing hobbies and pastimes, can lower stress levels and improve brain health in general.

Participating in social activities is another important barrier to Alzheimer's disease prevention. According to research, keeping an active social life, taking part in worthwhile conversations and activities, and having a solid support network can all assist to protect cognitive function and lower the risk of Alzheimer's disease. Building relationships with people helps us to feel fulfilled and purposeful, both of which are critical for brain health.

In addition to lifestyle modifications, there exist additional preventive measures that can be used to mitigate the likelihood of Alzheimer's disease. Cognitive stimulation is one such tool. Playing strategic games, learning a new language or instrument, solving puzzles, reading, and other mentally engaging activities can assist maintain cognitive function and lower the risk of cognitive decline. Furthermore, since chronic medical disorders like diabetes, hypertension, and high cholesterol raise the risk of Alzheimer's disease, it is critical to prioritise brain health by controlling these problems. Effective management of these disorders can be achieved by following prescribed treatment plans and scheduling routine check-ups with medical professionals.

In conclusion, millions of people worldwide suffer from the debilitating ailment known as Alzheimer's disease. There are a number of modifiable risk factors that can be addressed by lifestyle changes and preventive measures, however other risk factors, like age and heredity, cannot be modified. We may dramatically lower the risk of Alzheimer's disease by emphasising a nutritious diet, consistent exercise, restful sleep, stress management, social interaction, cognitive stimulation, and adequate medical care. In my capacity as a physician and health and wellness coach, I'm dedicated to providing people with the information and tools they need to take charge of their mental health and live free from the burden of Alzheimer's. When we work together, we can change things and provide future generations a better future.

Comorbidities and Complications

As a physician and health and wellness coach, I have direct experience with the myriad difficulties that people with Alzheimer's disease encounter. They deal with memory loss and cognitive decline in addition to being vulnerable to many comorbidities and problems that can worsen their symptoms and impair their general health. We shall examine these comorbidities and complications in detail in this subchapter, outlining their implications and providing management recommendations.

Depression is one of the most common comorbidities linked to Alzheimer's disease. Studies have indicated that the general population is not as likely to experience depression as people with Alzheimer's disease. This can be due to a number of things, such as the psychological effects of the illness itself, the social isolation that people with Alzheimer's disease sometimes face, and the difficulties associated with managing a progressing and incapacitating condition.

In addition to exacerbating depressive and hopeless feelings, depression in Alzheimer's patients exacerbates cognitive impairment. Increased agitation, impatience, and trouble performing daily tasks can result from it. Furthermore, because people with Alzheimer's disease may already be exhibiting comparable symptoms, like apathy and withdrawal, depression frequently goes undiagnosed in these patients.

It is consequently crucial to identify and treat depression in people with Alzheimer's disease. I regularly collaborate with my patients and their families as a health and wellness coach to recognise the warning symptoms of depression and put treatment plans in place. This entails maintaining social bonds, participating in activities that enhance wellbeing, and scheduling routine check-ins for mental health. In addition, a medical expert could advise treatment and medicines to treat depression and enhance the patient's and their caregivers' quality of life in general.

Another prevalent comorbidity that affects people with Alzheimer's disease is anxiety. It makes sense that having a neurological illness that progresses might cause anxiety and uneasiness. But anxiety can have a major negative effect on a person with Alzheimer's quality of life and ability to operate on a daily basis.

Restlessness, excessive worrying, and trouble focusing are common signs of anxiety. Additionally, it may result in bodily symptoms as dyspepsia, fast heartbeat, and dyspnea. These symptoms can worsen cognitive ageing and raise the chance of falls and accidents in those whose mobility is already impaired.

Alzheimer's sufferers need a multifaceted approach to anxiety management. To aid with anxiety symptoms, I use a variety of strategies in my practise, including mindfulness meditation, relaxation exercises, and cognitive-behavioral therapy. Anxiety triggers can also be reduced by establishing a quiet and orderly environment, encouraging consistency and predictability, and offering assurance and validation. To treat severe anxiety symptoms, doctors may give medication in some situations. However, these should be closely monitored and customised for each patient.

Another important comorbidity that can affect how Alzheimer's disease is managed is cardiovascular disease. Studies have demonstrated a robust association between heart health and cognitive abilities, with cardiovascular risk factors including high blood pressure, diabetes, and cholesterol putting people at an increased risk of Alzheimer's disease.

An individual's treatment and overall prognosis are considerably complicated when they have cardiovascular disease. Reduced blood supply to the brain can worsen cognitive ageing and accelerate the onset of Alzheimer's symptoms. Furthermore, the adverse effects of cardiovascular drugs, like diuretics and beta-blockers, may exacerbate memory loss and impair cognitive performance.

A comprehensive approach is required to handle the co-occurrence of Alzheimer's disease with cardiovascular disease. This entails following a heart-healthy diet, exercising frequently (to the extent that one is able), and keeping a careful eye on cholesterol and blood pressure readings. A medical practitioner should thoroughly assess medications to make sure they don't negatively impact cognitive function. Furthermore, for the proper coordination of the management of both illnesses, constant communication between the patient's primary care physician and the healthcare team is necessary.

To sum up, managing comorbidities and consequences is a crucial part of treating Alzheimer's disease. Conditions including anxiety, depression, and cardiovascular disease can impede overall well-being, worsen symptoms, and affect how quickly a disease progresses. In order to successfully treat these comorbidities and difficulties, as a medical doctor and health and wellness coach, I think that a comprehensive strategy that includes lifestyle changes, psychological support, and cooperation with a multidisciplinary team of experts is necessary. People with Alzheimer's can improve their quality of life and, to the best of their abilities, maintain their independence by learning about the effects of these disorders and putting management methods into place.

Caregiver Support and Resources

Support Networks:

Having a support system is crucial for caregivers of individuals with Alzheimer's disease. Family members, close friends, support networks, and medical professionals may fall under this category. Every one of these networks of support is essential in assisting caregivers in managing the particular difficulties they encounter.

Friends and relatives: Caregivers might benefit greatly from the emotional support provided by friends and family. They can share the caregiving duties, lend a helping hand, and lend a listening ear. It's critical for caregivers to express their needs and ask for help from those closest to them.

Support Teams: For caretakers, joining a support group can be quite beneficial. Support groups offer a secure environment where caregivers can talk about their experiences, trade advice and techniques, and get compassion and understanding from people going through comparable circumstances. Caretakers of people with Alzheimer's Disease can attend support groups organised by the Alzheimer's Association and nearby community centres.

Healthcare professionals: It's critical for caregivers to ask for advice and assistance from healthcare professionals. Physicians, nurses, and therapists can offer expert counsel, track an Alzheimer's patient's development, and support carers with a range of medical issues. Additionally, these experts are able to recommend and offer resources that are specifically catered to the needs of caregivers.

Respite Care Options:

It can be physically and mentally taxing to care for someone who has Alzheimer's disease. It's critical that caregivers put their own health first and take breaks when needed. Options for respite care offer caregivers short-term relief so they may rest and recover before taking up their caregiving duties again.

In-home respite care: This method is hiring a professional caregiver to help the primary caregiver temporarily. They can help with bathing, meal preparation, company, and other caring duties, providing the primary caregiver a break.

Adult day care centers: During the day, adult day care centres provide a secure and stimulating atmosphere for those with Alzheimer's disease. This gives caregivers peace of mind that their loved one is receiving excellent care, enabling them to pursue their own interests, take care of personal obligations, or just take a much-needed break. These facilities frequently offer a variety of programmes and activities created especially for people with cognitive disabilities.

Residential respite care: In certain situations, caregivers could need a lengthier break or have other obligations that need them to be gone for a prolonged period of time. With the assurance that their loved one is receiving round-the-clock care, residential respite care facilities give people with Alzheimer's Disease temporary housing. This enables their carers to take a much-needed vacation.

Strategies for Self-Care and Stress Management:

The emotional and physical toll of caring for someone with Alzheimer's disease can be high. It is imperative that caregivers put their own health first and take care of themselves. The following techniques can assist caregivers in stress management and wellbeing maintenance:

Self-care activities: Caregivers can regain their energy and lessen their stress by partaking in enjoyable and relaxing activities. This could be doing yoga or meditation, going for walks in the outdoors, reading, listening to music, or engaging in other interests and hobbies.

Good nutrition: Having a healthy diet is crucial to preserving your health. It is important for caregivers to have a diet rich in fruits, vegetables, whole grains, lean meats, and healthy fats. Staying well hydrated is also crucial.

Exercise: Frequent exercise has many positive effects on mental health in addition to maintaining physical health. Walking, jogging, swimming, or yoga are some of the activities caregivers can do to stay active and decompress.

Restful sleep: Getting enough sleep is essential for maintaining good physical and mental health. Getting enough sleep and creating a pattern that encourages peaceful sleep should be top priorities for caregivers.

Seeking emotional support: When they need it, caregivers should not be reluctant to ask for emotional help. This can entail reaching out to a dependable friend or relative, signing up for a support group, or getting therapy from a therapist with expertise in caregiver support.

Setting realistic expectations: High standards for themselves are common among caregivers, which can result in fatigue and feelings of inferiority or shame. Caregivers should always remind themselves that they are doing the best they can and establish reasonable expectations.

Taking breaks: Regular pauses are necessary for caregivers to refuel and tend to their own needs. The much-needed time off might be obtained by making use of respite care choices or asking for assistance from family and friends.

To sum up, caring for a person suffering from Alzheimer's disease may be both fulfilling and difficult. However, carers may make this trip easier if they have the correct support system, have access to options for respite care, and practise self-care and stress management. Caregivers can make sure they have the power and resilience to give their loved ones the best care possible by putting their own health first.

Chapter 2: Medical Management of Alzheimer's Disease

Current Medications for Alzheimer's Disease

It is crucial to remember that every person reacts to drugs differently, and that what works for one person might not work for another. Furthermore, a person's overall health and the stage of their sickness can affect how a medicine affects them. As a result, it's critical to collaborate closely with a medical expert to identify the best course of action in each unique situation.

Cholinesterase inhibitors and memantine are the two types of drugs that are frequently prescribed to treat Alzheimer's disease.

The most often given drugs for Alzheimer's disease are cholinesterase inhibitors, which include galantamine (Razadyne), rivastigmine (Exelon), and donepezil (Donecept, Aricept). These drugs function by raising the brain's concentration of acetylcholine, a neurotransmitter linked to memory and learning. These drugs work by preventing the breakdown of acetylcholine by the enzyme acetylcholinesterase, which helps enhance cognitive function.

There are two formulations of donepezil available: immediate-release and extended-release. One dose is administered daily for the immediate-release formulation and one dose is administered in the evening for the extended-release formulation. Rivastigmine comes in two forms: an oral patch that is worn topically once a day and an oral version that is taken twice a day with meals. There are three different forms of galantamine: tablet, extended-release capsule, and oral solution. The recommendations of the healthcare provider and the particular needs of the patient will determine the precise medicine kind and dosage.

Cholinesterase inhibitors may have adverse effects in addition to their possible benefits in treating cognitive problems. Dizziness, nausea, vomiting, diarrhoea, and appetite loss are a few of these adverse effects. Individuals and others who are caring for them should keep an eye out for any negative responses and notify their healthcare provider of them.

Another drug that is often used to treat Alzheimer's disease is memantine (Namenda). In contrast to cholinesterase inhibitors, which function by raising acetylcholine levels, memantine acts by controlling glutamate, another neurotransmitter. Although glutamate plays a role in memory and learning, too much of it can harm brain tissue.

There are two formulations of memantine available: immediate-release and extended-release. It is customary to take the immediate-release formulation twice day and the extended-release formulation once daily. Similar to cholinesterase inhibitors, memantine dose and type are based on the unique requirements of each patient.

Memantine adverse effects can include headache, constipation, dizziness, and disorientation. Although most of these side effects are transient and moderate, it's always vital to talk to a healthcare provider about any concerns you may have.

Apart from these treatments, several studies have investigated the possible advantages of other pharmaceuticals like statins, antidepressants, and nonsteroidal anti-inflammatory drugs (NSAIDs) in treating the cognitive symptoms of Alzheimer's disease. These trials have yielded inconsistent findings, though, and more investigation is required to determine their efficacy in this particular setting.

It is important to remember that taking medicine by itself cannot fully address the management of Alzheimer's disease. A comprehensive treatment strategy should include lifestyle changes such as social interaction, a balanced diet, frequent exercise, and enough sleep. Counseling and psychological strategies can also assist patients and their families in overcoming the psychological and emotional difficulties brought on by the illness.

In addition, supplementary and alternative therapies like music therapy, aromatherapy, and brain-training activities have shown some promise in enhancing cognitive performance and quality of life in Alzheimer's patients. To improve general well-being, these methods can be combined with conventional medication.

In summary, the goal of the drugs currently prescribed for Alzheimer's disease is to control cognitive symptoms while also reducing the illness's progression. The two most often given drugs are memantine and cholinesterase inhibitors, each of which has a unique mode of action and possible adverse effects. But it's crucial to understand that medicine is only one part of a thorough treatment programme that also needs to include counselling, supplemental therapies, and lifestyle changes. People with Alzheimer's disease and their families can maximise their quality of life and preserve as much independence as possible by managing the disease holistically.

Clinical Trials and Experimental Treatments

Clinical trials and experimental treatments for Alzheimer's disease have received a lot of attention in the last several years. These clinical studies are essential for expanding our knowledge of the illness, identifying novel therapeutic targets, and enhancing the lives of those who are affected by Alzheimer's and their loved ones. We will look at some of the most exciting new developments in the field and possible breakthroughs in this subchapter.

The creation of therapies that alter disease is one field with a lot of research activity. These therapies target the underlying degenerative mechanisms in the brain in an effort to reduce or even stop the progression of Alzheimer's disease. Monoclonal antibody therapy is one such experimental treatment that has demonstrated potential. One of the distinguishing features of Alzheimer's disease, amyloid-beta plaques, is intended to be precisely bound and eliminated by monoclonal antibodies. Researchers intend to slow down the disease's accompanying cognitive impairment by focusing on and removing these plaques. This treatment can effectively lower amyloid-beta plaques in the brain, according to certain clinical trials; nevertheless, more studies are required to completely evaluate how well it can enhance cognitive function.

The tau protein, which accumulates into tangles in the brains of Alzheimer's patients, is the subject of additional study. These tangles impede brain cell-to-brain transmission and worsen cognitive impairment. There are several experimental treatments being explored that target tau protein, such as small chemical inhibitors and vaccinations. The goal of these treatments is to encourage the removal of tau tangles that already exist or stop new ones from forming. Clinical trials have yielded promising preliminary results on the reduction of tau pathology. Currently, investigations are being conducted to assess the safety and effectiveness of these treatments.

In addition to therapies that alter the course of the disease, scientists are looking into interventions that can lessen the symptoms of Alzheimer's and enhance quality of life. Cognitive training is one such method. To preserve and enhance cognitive function, cognitive training entails intellectually demanding tasks including memory tests, puzzles, and computer-based applications. Numerous studies have demonstrated that cognitive training can help people with mild cognitive impairment and early-stage Alzheimer's disease improve their memory, concentration, and problem-solving abilities. Although additional investigation is required to establish the ideal frequency and length of cognitive training, it presents a viable option for non-pharmacological treatments.

Physical exercise has also drawn interest in the management of Alzheimer's disease, in addition to cognitive training. Frequent exercise has been demonstrated to improve cognitive performance in addition to physical health. Exercise is good for the brain because it increases blood flow to the brain, increases the synthesis of neurotrophic factors, and lowers inflammation. Studies looking into how exercise affects Alzheimer's disease have shown increases in mood, general well-being, and cognitive performance. These results bolster the idea that exercise is an essential part of managing Alzheimer's disease.

The application of dietary therapies for the management of Alzheimer's disease is the subject of additional investigation. Numerous studies have indicated that specific dietary regimens, including the MIND (Mediterranean-DASH Diet Intervention for Neurodegenerative Delay) or Mediterranean diet, may lower the risk of Alzheimer's disease and cognitive decline. These diets restrict processed meals, sugary snacks, and saturated fats while increasing the intake of fruits, vegetables, whole grains, lean protein, and healthy fats. According to the research, these dietary patterns include vital nutrients, anti-inflammatory agents, and antioxidants that support brain function and lower the risk of neurodegenerative illnesses. A promising approach to the management and prevention of Alzheimer's disease is to adopt a brain-healthy diet, while further study is required to clearly show a cause-and-effect relationship.

To sum up, research into Alzheimer's disease is still being advanced through clinical trials and experimental therapies. For those with Alzheimer's disease and their families, research and innovation in this sector provide hope in the form of disease-modifying medications and lifestyle treatments. I'm dedicated to keeping up with these developments as a medical doctor and health and wellness coach and implementing them into our all-encompassing treatment plan. We can provide people with Alzheimer's disease with a comprehensive plan for managing their disease and enjoying a higher quality of life by integrating alternative medicine, lifestyle changes, and experimental therapies.

Non-Pharmacological Interventions

One of the most important parts of controlling Alzheimer's disease is cognitive stimulation. The brain is an amazing organ that can grow and adapt incredibly well, even in the face of neurodegenerative diseases like Alzheimer's. Studies have demonstrated that mentally stimulating activities can assist people with Alzheimer's disease perform better and slow down their cognitive decline.

Programs for structured cognitive training are among the best ways to stimulate cognitive function. Participating in these programmes entails doing mental exercises that enhance cognitive performance. Puzzles, memory games, and problem-solving exercises, for instance, are frequently used to engage various brain regions and improve cognitive ability. These activities have long-term effects on brain health in addition to acute cognitive gains.

Exercise is a crucial component of non-pharmacological treatments for Alzheimer's disease. Frequent physical activity is crucial for preserving general health and wellbeing, and it is especially crucial for those who have Alzheimer's disease. Exercise improves cardiovascular health, increases cognitive function, and lowers the risk of chronic diseases, among many other advantages for the body and the brain.

Numerous studies have demonstrated the beneficial effects of exercise on cognitive performance in Alzheimer's disease patients. Specifically, aerobic exercise has been shown to enhance executive function, memory, and attention in this population. It is thought that physical activity improves cognitive performance by stimulating the formation of new nerve cells, releasing growth factors, and increasing blood supply to the brain.

Lifestyle changes are critical to controlling Alzheimer's disease, in addition to cognitive stimulation and physical exercise. Adopting a healthy lifestyle can significantly improve one's general state of wellbeing and possibly halt the disease's progression. The following significant lifestyle adjustments may be helpful for those suffering from Alzheimer's disease:

1. Balanced Diet: The nutrients required for optimal brain function are found in a diet rich in fruits, vegetables, whole grains, lean proteins, and healthy fats. This type of food is well-balanced. Studies have indicated that a plant-based, Mediterranean-style diet may help postpone the beginning of Alzheimer's disease and lower the risk of cognitive decline.

2. Adequate Sleep: Sleep is crucial for the health of the brain, and sleep difficulties are common in people with Alzheimer's disease. The quality of sleep and general cognitive performance can be enhanced by maintaining a regular sleep schedule and practising excellent sleep hygiene, which includes avoiding stimulants before bed and setting up a pleasant sleeping environment.

3. Stress Management: Prolonged stress may exacerbate Alzheimer's disease symptoms and has been connected to cognitive loss. Using stress-reduction strategies, such as mindfulness meditation, deep breathing exercises, and soothing pursuits, can aid in lowering stress levels and enhancing general wellbeing.

4. Social Engagement: It is imperative that people with Alzheimer's Disease maintain social contacts and participate in meaningful social activities. Social engagement boosts happiness, increases brain activity, and sharpens cognitive abilities. Engaging in social activities and being a member of a community that supports one another can improve one's overall quality of life and offer emotional support.

5. Intellectual Stimulation: Maintaining cognitive function and delaying cognitive decline can be achieved by continuing education and intellectually challenging activities. Reading, picking up a new skill or language, and taking up mentally demanding hobbies are all good ways to maintain the brain sharp and healthy.

It is crucial to remember that non-pharmacological therapies should be customised to each person with Alzheimer's Disease in order to fit their specific needs and preferences. Collaborating with a group of specialists from various health and wellness domains, such as physicians, dietitians, physiotherapists, and psychologists, can guarantee an all-encompassing and customised strategy for managing Alzheimer's disease.

In summary, non-pharmacological therapies such as physical activity, cognitive stimulation, and lifestyle changes are vital for the management of Alzheimer's disease. It has been demonstrated that these interventions improve general well-being, increase cognitive function, and may even reduce the disease's course. A comprehensive treatment strategy that includes these therapies can help people with Alzheimer's Disease live happy, fulfilling lives and preserve their cognitive abilities for as long as feasible.

Nutritional Approaches and Dietary Recommendations

The study of nutrition has advanced recently, and our knowledge of how dietary decisions affect human health has grown dramatically. It is now commonly acknowledged that for the best possible brain health, a diet rich in necessary nutrients and well-balanced. Certain dietary changes can significantly slow down the disease's course and improve cognitive performance in the context of Alzheimer's disease.

Nutrient-dense, complete foods are an essential part of a diet that promotes brain function. A variety of key elements, including vitamins, minerals, and antioxidants, are present in these foods and are crucial for preserving the health of the brain. A diet rich in fruits, vegetables, whole grains, lean proteins, and healthy fats—like those in nuts, avocados, and olive oil—has been linked to preventing Alzheimer's disease-related brain damage.

It's critical to pay attention to particular nutrients that have been demonstrated to enhance brain function in addition to emphasising entire foods. For example, omega-3 fatty acids have been associated with a lower incidence of cognitive decline and are necessary for the brain's optimal functioning. Walnuts and flaxseeds are good sources of omega-3 fatty acids, as are fatty fish like mackerel, salmon, and sardines. By incorporating these foods into your diet, you can get a sufficient amount of omega-3 fatty acids.

Antioxidants, such vitamins C and E, have also been demonstrated to be essential in shielding the brain from oxidative stress and lowering the likelihood of cognitive decline. You should include fruits and vegetables in your regular meals since they are great providers of antioxidants, especially berries, citrus fruits, and leafy greens.

Certain supplements, in addition to macro- and micronutrients, can help maintain brain health in Alzheimer's patients. But it's crucial to remember that supplements should never take the place of a healthy, balanced diet and should only ever be taken under a doctor's supervision. Certain supplements, such as ginkgo biloba, turmeric, and vitamin D, have demonstrated potential in promoting brain health. These supplements function by strengthening neuroplasticity, decreasing inflammation, and guarding against oxidative damage.

Gut health is another important component of diet that should not be disregarded in the context of managing Alzheimer's disease. A healthy gut flora is strongly correlated with optimal brain function, according to research. Known as the "gut-brain axis," it emphasises the reciprocal relationship in which the health of the gut and the brain influence each other.

It's crucial to incorporate a range of fibres in your diet to support gut health because they function as prebiotics and food for good gut flora. Fruits, vegetables, legumes, and whole grains are among the foods high in dietary fibre. Foods high in probiotics, like kefir, sauerkraut, kimchi, and yoghurt, can also help maintain a balanced gut microbiome.

It's crucial to take into account additional lifestyle choices that may have an impact on brain health in addition to food adjustments. For instance, studies have demonstrated that regular physical activity enhances cognitive performance and lowers the risk of Alzheimer's disease. Try to get in at least 150 minutes a week of moderate-to-intense exercise, including cycling, swimming, or brisk walking.

Another essential component of managing Alzheimer's disease is stress management. Prolonged stress can exacerbate Alzheimer's disease symptoms and contribute to cognitive impairment. Including stress-relieving activities in your daily routine, such as deep breathing exercises, moderate yoga, and mindfulness meditation, can help reduce stress and promote brain health.

Moreover, sufficient sleep is necessary for the brain to function at its best. Alzheimer's disease risk has been linked to irregular sleep patterns and sleep disturbances. To maintain brain health, aim for 7-8 hours of good sleep each night and create a regular sleep regimen.

In summary, it is impossible to overestimate the importance of nutrition in the management of Alzheimer's disease. People with Alzheimer's disease can slow down the advancement of the disease and enhance brain function by following certain nutrients and supplements, eating a brain-healthy diet that emphasises nutrient-dense whole foods, and placing a high priority on gut health. But it's important to keep in mind that a comprehensive management strategy for Alzheimer's disease should include other lifestyle changes like regular exercise, stress reduction, and enough sleep in addition to nutrition. Seeking advice from a medical expert or a certified dietitian can offer tailored direction and assistance to maximise your nutritional strategy for managing Alzheimer's disease.

Sleep and Alzheimer's Disease

Sleep. We all encounter this natural occurrence on a regular basis. As we close our eyes, our bodies go into a resting and rejuvenating condition and our minds become calmer. Our brains integrate memories, heal damaged tissue, and control a number of essential functions when we sleep. However, sleep can turn into a battlefield of uncertainty, unrest, and frustration for those who have Alzheimer's disease.

As a physician and health and wellness coach, I have worked with numerous individuals who have Alzheimer's disease-related sleep disturbances. These people frequently wake up in the middle of the night, move about a lot, and are more sleepy during the day. Moreover, studies have repeatedly demonstrated that sleep disorders might hasten the onset of Alzheimer's disease and worsen cognitive loss.

It is impossible to overstate the importance of sleep for cognitive performance. It has been discovered that sleep deprivation affects executive function, memory, and attention. It may result in issues with focus, solving problems, and making decisions. These cognitive deficiencies can be rather severe in Alzheimer's disease patients, which frequently leads to increased confusion, disorientation, and behavioural problems.

Thus, what steps may be taken to help people with Alzheimer's disease maintain better sleep hygiene? Let's explore a few methods that can lessen sleep disruptions and encourage higher-quality sleep.

The most important thing to remember is to stick to a regular sleep routine. Regular sleep is essential to the health of our bodies. Our internal clocks are trained to efficiently control our sleep-wake cycle by going to bed and getting up at regular times. People suffering from Alzheimer's disease can increase their chances of getting a good night's sleep by establishing a consistent sleep schedule.

It's also critical to create a sleeping-friendly environment. To encourage the best possible sleep environment, keep the bedroom quiet, cold, and dark. To block out distracting noises, think about utilising earplugs or white noise devices. A comfy pillow and bedding purchase can also have a big impact on how well you sleep.

Before going to bed, Alzheimer's patients can improve their ability to relax and get ready for sleep. Calm and tranquilly can be fostered by incremental muscular relaxation, progressive deep breathing techniques, and guided visualisation. Furthermore, it has been demonstrated that mindfulness meditation improves the quality of sleep for those who experience sleep disruptions.

Reducing alcohol and caffeine intake is crucial to improving the quality of your sleep. Both drugs have the ability to interfere with sleep cycles and cause nocturnal waking. Better sleep can be achieved by encouraging people with Alzheimer's disease to limit their intake of caffeinated beverages and abstain from alcohol close to bedtime.

It has been demonstrated that regular exercise enhances the quality of sleep for people of all ages. People with Alzheimer's disease may feel more exhausted at night and have an easier time falling asleep if they exercise moderately during the day. To avoid overstimulating the body right before bed, it's crucial to make sure exercise is done earlier in the day.

Establishing a nightly wind-down regimen can help the body recognise when it's time to unwind and get ready for sleep. This regimen may involve things like reading a book, having a warm bath, or enjoying some relaxing music. Individuals with Alzheimer's Disease can teach their bodies to link certain activities with sleep by developing a regular winding-down regimen.

It might be essential to speak with a healthcare provider if sleep difficulties continue after trying these solutions. People with Alzheimer's disease can treat their sleep disturbances using a variety of drugs and therapies. Medication should, however, always be used as a last resort and in conjunction with other non-pharmacological interventions, it is crucial to keep in mind.

In conclusion, sleep problems can have a major effect on an Alzheimer's disease patient's cognitive abilities and general well-being. We can lessen the impact of sleep disturbances and enhance the quality of life for these people by emphasising the improvement of sleep hygiene. There are many tactics that can be used, such as making a sleep-friendly environment, practising relaxation techniques, and scheduling regular sleep times. It is my goal that the material in this subchapter will be of great use to those who are caring for someone who has Alzheimer's disease. By working together, we can enable people living with Alzheimer's disease to develop sound sleeping practises and improve their quality of life.

Managing Behavioral and Psychological Symptoms

Knowing the underlying causes of behavioural and psychological symptoms in Alzheimer's disease is crucial to addressing them. These symptoms are frequently brought on by the disease's alterations to the brain, while they can also be impacted by other elements including pain, side effects from medications, or environmental influences. Alzheimer's patients can have better quality of life and more effective symptom management by recognising and treating these underlying causes.

Those suffering from Alzheimer's disease frequently experience agitation, which is typified by restlessness, impatience, and emotional anguish. This can be tough for the person with the disability as well as their carers because it frequently results in communication problems and elevated stress levels. Establishing a tranquil and comfortable setting is one method of agitation management. This can be accomplished by reducing background noise and other distractions, sticking to a regular schedule, and creating a cosy and familiar environment. Reducing agitation and promoting relaxation can also be achieved by getting the person involved in activities they enjoy, including light exercise or music.

Another behavioural characteristic of Alzheimer's disease that can be upsetting for the patient and their caretakers is aggression. It frequently results from frustration or confusion and might take the form of verbal or physical hostility. Safety for the aggressor and anyone around them must come first while handling aggressiveness. This can entail clearing out anything that might be used as a weapon and establishing a tranquil, safe space. Another way to defuse a situation is to offer a distraction or refocus the person's attention on something else. In certain situations, controlling aggression may also benefit from drug administration and medical advice.

A typical psychological symptom of Alzheimer's disease is depression, which is frequently brought on by social isolation, cognitive decline, and loss of independence. It's critical to recognise the telltale symptoms of depression, which include thoughts of hopelessness, indifference in activities, changes in eating or sleep patterns, and chronic melancholy. In order to effectively manage depression in people with Alzheimer's disease, a multifaceted strategy is frequently required. This could involve social interaction to create a feeling of purpose and belonging, pharmaceutical management to reduce symptoms, and therapy or counselling to address the emotional and psychological components. Additionally, mood and general well-being can benefit from leading a healthy lifestyle that includes frequent exercise, a balanced diet, and social engagement.

Another prevalent psychological symptom of Alzheimer's disease is anxiety, which is typified by restlessness, worry, and emotions of fear. Physical symptoms like elevated heart rate, dyspnea, and upset stomach are common manifestations of it. In order to manage anxiety in people with Alzheimer's disease, one should establish a peaceful and consistent environment, offer comfort and support, and take part in stress-relieving activities like mindfulness exercises or deep breathing exercises. In certain situations, managing medication and seeking medical advice can also be helpful in reducing anxiety symptoms.

It's critical to keep in mind that every person with Alzheimer's Disease is different and may react differently to different tactics while managing behavioural and psychological symptoms. Depending on the preferences and skills of the individual, treatments may need to be adjusted and modified as needed. Involving a multidisciplinary team of professionals from various wellness and health domains can also offer a thorough method of treating these symptoms. This may include experts who may provide direction and assistance in meeting the many requirements of people with Alzheimer's Disease, such as psychologists, social workers, occupational therapists, and dietitians.

In summary, treating behavioural and psychological symptoms of Alzheimer's disease necessitates a comprehensive strategy that takes into account the underlying causes and offers customised symptom management techniques. We can successfully control agitation, anger, depression, and anxiety in people with the disease by establishing a comfortable and familiar atmosphere, encouraging participation in worthwhile activities, and attending to emotional and psychological well-being. Involving a multidisciplinary team of professionals can also offer comprehensive and customised help to people with Alzheimer's disease and those who care for them. Individuals suffering from Alzheimer's Disease can achieve greater well-being and a higher quality of life with the appropriate techniques and assistance.

End-of-Life Care and Palliative Approaches

Chapter Eight: End-of-Life Care and Palliative Approaches

"The experience of losing a loved one to Alzheimer's disease can be extremely distressing and traumatic. It is our responsibility as medical professionals to offer the patient and their family comfort, support, and high-quality treatment during this trying time. This chapter will cover hospice care, advance care planning, and methods for maintaining comfort and dignity in the latter stages of the disease. It will also include palliative care for people with Alzheimer's disease."

Section One: Advance Care Planning

"It is crucial that patients and their families talk about and decide on their future care at the early stages of Alzheimer's disease. We call this advance care planning. It entails planning ahead and selecting the care and therapies that an individual would like in the later stages of their illness, when they might not be able to express their preferences."

1.1 Understanding the Importance of Advance Care Planning

"By expressing their preferences for medical care, living arrangements, and end-of-life care, people can make sure their intentions are fulfilled and respected by engaging in advance care planning. It also lessens the load for family members who might later have to make tough choices."

1.2 Initiating the Conversation

"It can be difficult to start talking about future care, but it is important that people with Alzheimer's disease and their families have these conversations as soon as possible. In my capacity as a healthcare professional, I promote direct and honest communication, fostering a safe environment in which patients and their families can share their worries, anxieties, and wishes."

1.3 Determining the Patient's Wishes

"We discuss different scenarios and treatment alternatives with patients during the advance care planning process to make sure their desires are recognised and documented. This entails talking about end-of-life desires, healthcare proxy designations, and durable power of attorney for healthcare, among other crucial decisions."

Section Two: Hospice Care

"Hospice care is a vital resource when curative treatments are no longer effective in the later stages of Alzheimer's disease. Hospice offers comprehensive care and assistance to patients suffering from severe dementia, emphasising emotional stability, pain control, and comfort."

2.1 Transitioning to Hospice Care

"It would be prudent to think about switching to hospice care when the patient's life expectancy is estimated to be six months or less due to the progression of the disease. The patient, their family, and the medical staff collaborate to make this choice."

2.2 The Hospice Care Team

"Hospice care is provided by a group of committed specialists with specialised training in end-of-life care. It is a multidisciplinary approach. With their individual specialties and talents, doctors, nurses, social workers, spiritual care providers, and volunteers usually make up this team."

2.3 Providing Comfort and Dignity

"Hospice care is primarily concerned with giving the patient comfort and dignity. This entails providing adequate pain and symptom management, guaranteeing emotional and spiritual support, and fostering a tranquil and serene atmosphere. Improving the patient's and their loved ones' quality of life during this difficult period is the aim."

Section Three: Strategies for Ensuring Comfort and Dignity

"Healthcare providers can use a number of techniques, such as advance care planning and hospice care, to guarantee the comfort and dignity of patients with Alzheimer's disease as the illness progresses.

These tactics take into account one's mental, emotional, and physical well."

3.1 Physical Comfort

"Ensuring physical comfort is crucial while providing end-of-life care. This entails managing pain, helping with personal hygiene and care, and making sure the patient's physical surroundings promote safety and comfort. Skin integrity, mobility, and nourishment are given careful consideration."

3.2 Emotional and Psychological Support

"Support for both emotional and psychological needs is critical to the wellbeing of people with Alzheimer's disease and their family. This could entail providing therapeutic interventions including art therapy, music therapy, and memory therapy. Furthermore, patients and their families can vent their feelings and find comfort in shared experiences through counselling and support groups."

3.3 Non-Pharmacological Approaches

"In addition to medication, non-pharmacological methods can be helpful in the palliative care of patients with Alzheimer's disease. These could include using sensory stimulation to encourage relaxation and wellbeing, aromatherapy, massage treatment, mindfulness and relaxation techniques, and more."

Chapter Eight Summary:

"This chapter has covered the significance of advance care planning, the function of hospice care in providing consolation and support, and methods for encouraging the physical, mental, and spiritual well-being of Alzheimer's patients as the disease progresses. Through the integration of a comprehensive strategy into end-of-life care, we can assist patients and their families in enduring this trying time with grace and empathy."

My team and I are committed to giving people with Alzheimer's Disease full care as a medical doctor and health and fitness coach. We work to improve the lives of our patients and their families at every stage of the disease by implementing lifestyle changes, creating individualised treatment plans, and emphasising emotional health. By working together, we can turn the difficulty presented by Alzheimer's disease into a chance for development, comprehension, and compassion.

The Role of Technology in Alzheimer's Disease Management

In the long run, assistive technology has been a mainstay in the treatment of Alzheimer's disease. These gadgets are made to aid people with everyday tasks and keep their independence for as long as feasible. One such gadget that the person with Alzheimer's disease can wear is a GPS tracking device. With the use of this gadget, caretakers can monitor their loved one's location, increasing safety and bringing comfort. Furthermore, there are smart home technologies that can be included into an Alzheimer's patient's living space. By automating actions like locking doors, turning off appliances, and regulating temperature, these technologies lower the chance of accidents and improve the quality of life for those who suffer from the illness.

Digital tools have been shown to be effective aids for managing Alzheimer's disease. People who struggle with communication, memory loss, or cognitive disability can benefit from a variety of apps. For example, there are apps that track daily routines, remind users to take their meds, and provide memory games to improve cognitive function. These resources help people with Alzheimer's Disease feel engaged and empowered in addition to helping them maintain their independence.

New technologies are completely changing the field of managing Alzheimer's disease. Virtual reality is one such technology that has demonstrated significant promise in enhancing cognitive function and lowering agitation in Alzheimer's patients. Virtual reality experiences have the power to take people to new places, arousing their senses and providing a mental workout. Additionally, wearable technology is being developed to track vital signs, give real-time feedback, and identify behavioural changes that might be symptoms of Alzheimer's disease progression. These technologies not only raise the standard of care but also give medical professionals useful information with which to make treatment plan decisions.

Not only has technology affected those who have Alzheimer's disease, but also those who care for them. It can be physically and emotionally taxing to care for someone who has Alzheimer's disease, which frequently leads to high levels of stress and burnout. Thank goodness, technology has intervened to ease some of these difficulties. Apps designed to assist caregivers are available and offer tools, advice, and techniques for handling the day-to-day challenges of providing care for an individual with Alzheimer's disease. Support groups, medication reminders, and even virtual consultations with medical professionals are all provided by these apps, guaranteeing that caregivers will always have access to the assistance they require.

Technology is unquestionably essential for managing Alzheimer's disease, but it's important to remember that technology can never take the place of a human touch. Technology use ought to be viewed as an addition to conventional therapies and interventions. It can undoubtedly improve the quality of life for those who have Alzheimer's disease and those who care for them, but it shouldn't take the place of the knowledge, care, and compassion that are the cornerstones of holistic healthcare.

In summary, technology's role in managing Alzheimer's disease is always changing and growing. Emerging technology, digital tools, and assistive gadgets are transforming how we provide care and assistance to people with the illness. Technologies such as virtual reality and GPS monitoring devices provide creative ways to improve safety, autonomy, and cognitive performance. Technology also helps caregivers; caregiver support applications offer essential tools and assistance to overcome the difficulties of caring for an individual with Alzheimer's disease. But it's crucial to keep in mind that technology should never take the place of the interpersonal relationships that are crucial to healthcare. We can genuinely enable people with Alzheimer's disease and those who care for them to lead happy and meaningful lives by incorporating technology into a holistic approach to care.

Chapter 3: Holistic Approaches to Alzheimer's Disease Management

Mindfulness and Meditation

This chapter delves into the topics of mindfulness and meditation, examining the significant impact these practises have on people living with Alzheimer's disease. We will talk about these activities' immense potential for improving overall well-being, stress reduction, and cognitive function. People suffering from Alzheimer's Disease can improve their quality of life and start a journey of self-discovery and recovery by adding mindfulness and meditation into their everyday routines.

Stress Reduction:

It can be frightening and overwhelming to live with Alzheimer's disease, for both the afflicted person and their loved ones. Stress levels can grow from the ongoing fight to maintain cognitive function, traverse memories, and adjust to a constantly changing reality. Prolonged stress can exacerbate Alzheimer's disease symptoms and have a negative impact on one's physical and mental well-being.

Thankfully, mindfulness and meditation offer a break from the stress storm. Through the practise of living in the present moment, people with Alzheimer's Disease can temporarily escape the grip of tension and anxiety by cultivating a sense of serenity and tranquillity. The mind is able to free itself from the hold of previous memories and future worries by practising guided breathing techniques and focused concentration.

Additionally, studies have demonstrated the benefits of mindfulness and meditation in controlling the body's stress response system. Hormones like cortisol are released as a result of ongoing stress, and they can be harmful to one's general health and cognitive abilities. Nonetheless, it has been discovered that engaging in mindfulness and meditation practises lowers cortisol levels, encouraging relaxing and reestablishing physical and mental balance. In addition to directly enhancing wellbeing, this stress reduction helps those who have Alzheimer's disease perform cognitively better.

Cognitive Function:

The gradual loss of cognitive function is one of the biggest problems that people with Alzheimer's Disease have to deal with. Among this crippling condition's signature symptoms are memory loss, difficulties solving problems, and poor decision-making abilities. However, there is some hope in the form of mindfulness and meditation when it comes to cognitive deterioration.

The beneficial effects of mindfulness and meditation on cognitive function have been shown in numerous studies. It has been demonstrated that these techniques increase cognitive flexibility overall, improve memory, and improve focus and concentration. People with Alzheimer's disease may be able to slow down the cognitive loss that comes with the disease by practising mindfulness and meditation on a daily basis. This will help them remember things better, build relationships, and have meaningful discussions.

Furthermore, the psychological discomfort that frequently accompanies cognitive loss might be lessened with the use of mindfulness and meditation. With these activities, frustration, uncertainty, and worry can be greatly minimised, resulting in a greater sense of peace and clarity for those with Alzheimer's disease. People who have achieved this increased emotional well-being are better able to direct their mental energies into endeavours that promote personal development and exploration, which in turn enhances cognitive performance.

Overall Well-being:

When someone is diagnosed with Alzheimer's disease, they frequently experience feelings of hopelessness and despair. It can be quite upsetting to gradually lose one's sense of self and memories. But finding purpose in the middle of turmoil and accepting the present moment is possible with the help of mindfulness and meditation.

A strong sense of self-awareness and self-compassion is fostered by practising mindfulness and meditation. Alzheimer's patients can learn to accept their current situation with grace and composure by developing an attitude of acceptance and non-judgment. These activities help people to appreciate the present and find joy in even the most mundane times rather than mourning the passing of memories.

Moreover, the advantages of mindfulness and meditation go beyond the lives of those who have Alzheimer's disease. Because they too can benefit from decreased stress, improved wellbeing, and increased emotional resilience, caregivers and loved ones can attest to the transformational potential of these activities. In the context of Alzheimer's disease, the ripple effects of mindfulness and meditation extend beyond personal borders and promote a supportive and understanding community.

To sum up, mindfulness and meditation have a great deal of potential for those with Alzheimer's disease. In the face of cognitive loss, these techniques provide a haven of serenity by lowering stress, boosting wellbeing, and restoring cognitive function. Through the integration of mindfulness and meditation into their daily routines, those diagnosed with Alzheimer's Disease can experience a profound journey of self-exploration and find comfort in the face of obstacles. I strongly endorse these methods as helpful aids in the management of Alzheimer's Disease as a medical practitioner and health and wellness coach. As we begin our journey towards holistic well-being and mastery of managing Alzheimer's disease, let's embrace the power of the present moment.

Yoga and Tai Chi for Brain Health

Historical Timeline:

Prior to discussing the particular advantages of yoga and tai chi for brain health, it's critical to comprehend the background information on these age-old traditions. Since its inception over 5,000 years ago in ancient India, yoga has gained popularity due to its all-encompassing approach to mental and physical health. In contrast, tai chi originated in ancient China over 2,000 years ago and is based on martial arts. It emphasises the harmony between the mind and body.

Due to their profound effects on mental and cognitive health, as well as their physical benefits, yoga and tai chi have become more popular worldwide. These techniques have long been known to be useful for raising feelings of calmness, lowering stress levels, and improving concentration.

Scientific Research:

Studies have begun to clarify the particular advantages of yoga and tai chi for maintaining brain health, particularly in those suffering from Alzheimer's disease. These activities have been shown in numerous studies to have positive impacts on memory, cognitive function, and general mental health.

A University of California, Los Angeles (UCLA) study found that practising yoga on a daily basis can enhance brain function in people with mild cognitive impairment, which is frequently seen as an early sign of Alzheimer's disease. In comparison to individuals who did not practise yoga, the researchers discovered that those who regularly practised yoga showed notable gains in their ability to concentrate, pay attention, and remember things.

Furthermore, the effects of tai chi on people with Alzheimer's disease were examined in a study that was published in the Journal of Alzheimer's Disease. Researchers discovered that practising tai chi increased individuals' overall quality of life, reduced their anxiety and despair, and improved their cognitive function. These results demonstrate tai chi's potential as a non-pharmacological treatment for Alzheimer's disease symptoms.

Poses, Movements, and Breathing Techniques:

Now, let's explore the specific poses, movements, and breathing techniques that can be beneficial for individuals with Alzheimer's Disease.

Yoga Poses:

1. Vrikshasana (Tree Pose): This standing position enhances concentration and balance. It is standing on one leg with the other foot planted firmly on the inside thigh of the standing leg. This position improves stability and focus, which improves cognitive performance.

2. Matsyasana (Fish Pose): This is a reclining backbend stance that stimulates the brain and extends the neck, spine, and chest. Additionally, it lowers tension and straightens posture, both of which enhance cognitive performance.

3. Nadi Shodhana Pranayama (Alternate Nostril Breathing): Using this breathing method, you close one nostril with your thumb while inhaling through the other, then exhale through the other. It balances the left and right hemispheres of the brain, eases anxiety, and encourages mental clarity.

Tai Chi Movements:

1. Cloud Hands: Focus is enhanced and mental stimulation is provided by this soft, flowing motion. It entails transferring weight from one leg to the other while rotating the arms in recurring circular rhythms.

2. Brush Knee and Twist Step: This exercise entails stepping forward on one foot, turning the torso, and brushing your arms together. It enhances mental clarity, balance, and coordination.

3. Standing Like a Tree: Standing with the feet shoulder-width apart, knees slightly bent, and arms raised as though embracing a tree,

this is a straightforward yet effective position. It fosters focus, serenity, and a feeling of stability.

For those suffering from Alzheimer's disease, a combination of certain yoga poses, tai chi movements, and particular breathing exercises can be quite beneficial. Frequent practise can improve mental health generally by lowering stress and anxiety, increasing focus and memory, and enhancing cognitive function.

Conclusion:

Finally, research indicates that tai chi and yoga can significantly improve cognitive function and brain health in Alzheimer's patients. The scientific study and historical background of these practises attest to their efficaciousness in augmenting mental well-being, mitigating stress, and improving focus. People with Alzheimer's Disease can significantly enhance their memory, cognitive function, and overall quality of life by regularly practising particular poses, movements, and breathing techniques. To guarantee safety and customise the practise to each person's needs and skills, it is crucial to speak with a certified instructor. Let's embrace the potential of tai chi and yoga as important tools for managing Alzheimer's disease together.

Art Therapy and Creative Expression

Painting and Drawing:

Painting and drawing are two of the most popular types of art therapy for people with Alzheimer's disease. These creative pursuits activate several brain regions, enhancing cognitive function and enhancing memory, focus, and problem-solving abilities. People feel more in charge and have more agency when they choose their colours, mix paints, and handle brushes; this increases their self-confidence and self-esteem.

For those suffering from Alzheimer's disease, painting and drawing have emotional advantages in addition to cognitive ones. It provides a release and outlet for their sentiments by enabling them to communicate their experiences and emotions nonverbally. Making something lovely and meaningful improves the emotional well-being of people with Alzheimer's disease by giving them a sense of accomplishment and purpose.

Music Therapy:

Music therapy is an additional efficacious art therapy modality for patients diagnosed with Alzheimer's Disease. The brain is profoundly affected by music, which stimulates neural connections and evokes emotional memories. According to studies, people with Alzheimer's disease frequently have musical memory preservation, which means they are still able to remember and appreciate music from the past. People with Alzheimer's Disease can connect with their emotional experiences and feel happy, cosy, and nostalgic by listening to and singing along to beloved tunes.

Alzheimer's patients may benefit cognitively from music therapy as well. Playing an instrument or singing calls for the use of a number of cognitive abilities, such as coordination, attention, and memory. People with Alzheimer's disease can exercise and increase these cognitive capacities by active participation in music therapy, which can assist to maintain or improve general cognitive function.

Other Artistic Mediums:

For those with Alzheimer's Disease, art therapy can use a variety of artistic mediums in addition to painting, drawing, and music. For instance, creating sculptures with clay or other tactile materials is a sensory-rich activity that activates the hands and the brain. This tactile interaction helps people relax and reduce stress in addition to improving cognitive performance.

Another common kind of art therapy for those with Alzheimer's disease is photography and collage-making. Through these exercises, people are encouraged to investigate their surroundings, seize important moments, and turn their memories into tangible artefacts. People with Alzheimer's disease can stimulate different parts of their brains and encourage cognitive stimulation and creative expression by interacting with visual stimuli.

Conclusion:

Using creative expression and art therapy can be a potent and successful way to control Alzheimer's disease. Several brain regions are activated by painting, drawing, music, and other artistic mediums, which boosts emotional health and cognitive performance. Through these artistic endeavours, people with Alzheimer's disease can discover their inner creative selves, find happiness, meaning, and a way to express themselves, as well as have fulfilling and connected moments. As a physician and health and wellness advisor, I have personally seen how art therapy may significantly improve the lives of those who have Alzheimer's disease. A complete plan for managing Alzheimer's disease might include art therapy to help people maximise their overall quality of life, emotional health, and cognitive performance.

Herbal Remedies and Supplements

Before getting into the particular herbs and supplements, it's critical to understand that, despite any potential advantages, they are not intended to take the place of traditional medical therapies for Alzheimer's disease. Rather, they can support and strengthen current therapeutic approaches, assisting in the management of symptoms and raising general quality of life.

Gingko Biloba is one herb whose potential advantages for brain health have drawn a lot of attention recently. This herb, which is made from the leaves of the gingko tree, is said to improve memory and cognitive performance. Gingko Biloba may lessen cognitive decline and enhance cognitive performance in Alzheimer's patients, according to a number of studies. It is crucial to remember that these studies' findings have been conflicting, and additional investigation is required to draw firm conclusions.

Another popular herbal therapy for managing Alzheimer's disease is curcumin, which is the active ingredient in turmeric. Due to its well-known anti-inflammatory and antioxidant qualities, curcumin may be able to lessen inflammation and shield the brain from oxidative damage. Supplementing with curcumin may help people with Alzheimer's disease with their memory and cognitive function, according to several studies. It is crucial to remember that curcumin has a restricted bioavailability, which means that the body does not absorb it quickly. It is frequently advised to consume curcumin with black pepper or in a supplement form that has been specially developed for increased bioavailability in order to promote absorption.

Apart from Gingko Biloba and Curcumin, a number of additional herbs and supplements have demonstrated potential in the management of Alzheimer's disease. These consist of:

1. Ashwagandha: Ashwagandha is an adaptogenic herb that comes from the root of the Withania somnifera plant and is said to lower

stress and enhance cognitive performance. According to preliminary research, ashwagandha may improve memory and cognitive function in Alzheimer's patients as well as provide neuroprotective advantages.

2. Bacopa Monnieri: Bacopa Monnieri, also known as Brahmi, is a herb that has been employed for its cognitive-enhancing qualities in ancient Ayurvedic medicine. Bacopa Monnieri may help with memory and cognitive function, according to a number of studies, which makes it a potentially helpful supplement for managing Alzheimer's disease.

3. Omega-3 Fatty Acids: Omega-3 fatty acids, which are abundant in fatty fish like salmon and mackerel, have been well researched for their possible advantages to brain function. Supplementing with omega-3 fatty acids may enhance cognitive performance and lower the likelihood of cognitive decline in people suffering from Alzheimer's disease, according to several studies. It's usually advised to take fish oil supplements or include foods high in omega-3 fatty acids.

4. Vitamin E: Vitamin E is a potent antioxidant that may help shield the brain from oxidative damage. Supplementing with vitamin E may improve cognitive performance and decrease the progression of Alzheimer's disease, according to certain studies. It is crucial to remember that excessive vitamin E intake may raise the risk of bleeding, particularly in people who are using blood thinners.

Although these vitamins and herbal therapies have potential for managing Alzheimer's disease, it is important to use caution when using them. Before beginning any new therapy or supplement, always get medical advice, especially if you have a pre-existing medical condition or are on any drugs that might interfere with these herbs and supplements.

It's also critical to keep in mind that each person may respond differently to supplements and herbal therapies in terms of their efficacy. One person's solution might not be another's. Discovering the ideal blend of herbs and vitamins for you may need some trial and error.

Finally, the realm of herbal therapies and supplements for managing Alzheimer's disease has been covered in this section. Although there is hope that these non-traditional therapy approaches can improve cognitive function and slow down cognitive decline, it is crucial to proceed cautiously and seek advice from a healthcare provider. Through the integration of evidence-based guidelines and customised tactics, people can leverage the potential advantages of herbal medicines and supplements to enhance their general health and wellness in the context of managing Alzheimer's disease.

Acupuncture and Traditional Chinese Medicine

Qi, or life energy, is stimulated through the use of tiny needles to certain body locations in acupuncture, an age-old therapy based in Traditional Chinese Medicine (TCM). Alzheimer's disease, according to TCM principles, is brought on by an imbalance in the body's energy flow, specifically in the brain. Acupuncture seeks to ease symptoms and improve general health by reestablishing the harmonious flow of Qi.

Enhancing cognitive function is one of the main advantages of acupuncture for managing Alzheimer's disease. Empirical studies have demonstrated the potential of acupuncture to augment cerebral blood flow, improve neurotransmitter functionality, and stimulate neuronal regeneration. The brain regions afflicted by Alzheimer's disease can be targeted and their regeneration and healing aided by activating particular acupuncture sites.

Acupuncture has a number of additional possible benefits for people with Alzheimer's Disease in addition to enhancing cognitive function. Stress and anxiety are frequent in people with the illness, and it can help lessen these. Research indicates that acupuncture can control the release of stress hormones while also fostering a feeling of calm and wellness.

Additionally, acupuncture helps those who have Alzheimer's disease sleep better. Patients with Alzheimer's disease frequently experience sleep disturbances, which exacerbates daytime weariness and impairs cognition. Acupuncture can help normalise sleep patterns and encourage restful sleep by addressing the underlying imbalances that lead to sleep disorders.

Acupuncture's capacity to decrease the disease's course is another crucial feature in the treatment of Alzheimer's. Research has demonstrated that acupuncture helps prevent the build-up of beta-amyloid plaques, which are indicative of Alzheimer's disease and have a role in the destruction of brain tissue. Acupuncture may help maintain cognitive function and prevent symptoms from getting worse by slowing down the buildup of these plaques.

Our all-encompassing strategy for managing Alzheimer's disease includes traditional Chinese herbal therapy as a crucial component. Based on each person's particular pattern of imbalances and symptoms, herbal treatments are chosen with great care. The goals of these treatments are to promote general health and wellbeing as well as bodily harmony.

"Kidney" system tonification and nourishment is one of the main tenets of traditional Chinese herbal treatment. According to TCM, memory and cognitive function are intimately related to the kidney system, which controls the brain. Alzheimer's disease can be slowed down in its progression and brain health can be supported by nourishing the kidney system with suitable herbal treatments.

Our strategy for managing Alzheimer's disease includes not only herbal medications but also dietary changes. The value of eating healthy foods that promote brain health is emphasised in traditional Chinese medicine. Foods high in antioxidants, such as leafy greens, berries, nuts, and seeds, are thought to improve cognitive function and may even prevent the onset of Alzheimer's disease.

We include a variety of self-care practises and coping mechanisms in our Alzheimer's Disease management programme in addition to acupuncture, herbal therapy, and dietary adjustments. These consist of cognitive activities, mindfulness exercises, stress management strategies, and meditation. By integrating various modalities, we provide our patients a comprehensive strategy for addressing Alzheimer's disease symptoms and enhancing general wellbeing.

Importantly, standard medical treatment for Alzheimer's disease should be combined with complementary therapies such as acupuncture and traditional Chinese medicine. By offering patients more assistance in controlling their symptoms and enhancing their quality of life, these modalities can augment the efficacy of conventional care.

To sum up, acupuncture and traditional Chinese medicine are effective therapies for Alzheimer's disease. They are an integral part of an all-encompassing therapy approach for people with Alzheimer's Disease because of their capacity to improve cognitive performance, reduce stress and anxiety, improve sleep quality, and delay the disease's progression. Our patients' general health and well-being have significantly improved as a result of incorporating these modalities into our management strategy for Alzheimer's disease.

Animal-Assisted Therapy

Since it has been used for millennia, animal-assisted therapy has shown to be a successful therapeutic strategy for a variety of neurological and mental illnesses. As a physician and health and wellness coach who is passionate about providing holistic healthcare, I have seen firsthand the enormous benefits that therapy animals can provide to those who are suffering from Alzheimer's disease. In my years of experience, I have witnessed the many therapeutic advantages that these creatures offer, which not only enhance happiness and camaraderie but also general well-being.

The history of animal therapy dates back to the Egyptians, who integrated animals into their ceremonies after realising the therapeutic value of animals. The idea of animal-assisted therapy came to light in more modern times, during World War II, when it was noted that troops who engaged with therapy dogs reported feeling less stressed and having better mental health. Since then, more and more research has been done on the therapeutic advantages of animals, which has resulted in the creation of official programmes for animal-assisted therapy.

Pets used as therapy animals, usually dogs or cats, are hand-picked and taught to engage with those suffering from Alzheimer's disease. To guarantee that they are well-mannered, compliant, and at ease in a variety of hospital environments, these animals go through specialised training. An atmosphere that is peaceful and judgment-free is fostered by the use of animals in treatment, which is especially important for those suffering from Alzheimer's disease who may experience anxiety or confusion.

The potential of animal-assisted treatment to lower stress is one of its main benefits for those with Alzheimer's disease. Alzheimer's patients frequently experience agitation and anxiety, which makes daily tasks difficult for them. Because therapy animals offer a sense of protection and comfort, their presence can help reduce these symptoms. According to research, spending time with animals lowers cortisol levels and releases oxytocin, which lessens stress and enhances emotional health.

Animal-assisted therapy has been shown to enhance the mood of Alzheimer's patients in addition to lowering stress. Many people who have this illness frequently struggle with despair and other unpleasant feelings. Therapy animals' unwavering compassion and love have the power to arouse emotions of contentment and happiness. The relationship that develops between the therapy animal and the Alzheimer's patient can lift their spirits and provide them with happy moments that might otherwise be hard to come by.

Furthermore, for those suffering from Alzheimer's disease, animal-assisted therapy helps improve social relationships. This illness frequently results in social distancing and retreat from close relationships, which lowers general social abilities. When used as a social catalyst, therapy animals can inspire people to interact and have conversations with both the animal and its human handlers. This kind of engagement can assist rekindle a feeling of interpersonal connection, enhance communication skills, and develop cognitive capacities.

Moreover, patients with Alzheimer's Disease may see improvements in their physical health as a result of animal-assisted therapy. It has been discovered that the presence of therapy animals lowers heart rate and blood pressure, improving cardiovascular health. Furthermore, soft pet care and grooming can assist people with Alzheimer's disease maintain or even enhance their physical abilities by enhancing their motor skills and dexterity.

Studies have repeatedly shown how effective animal-assisted therapy is in enhancing the quality of life for those who suffer from Alzheimer's disease. In an Alzheimer's Disease study that was published in the Journal of Geriatric Psychiatry, participants who participated in therapy animal sessions reported feeling less stressed, more socially engaged, and having better overall health. Another study that was published in the Journal of the American Geriatrics Society discovered that people with Alzheimer's disease who interacted with therapy animals showed improvements in their cognitive abilities as well as a decrease in their depressive symptoms.

To sum up, there are a lot of therapeutic advantages to animal-assisted therapy for Alzheimer's patients. The presence of therapy animals has a favourable effect on physical health, happiness, social relationships, and stress reduction. In my capacity as a physician and health and wellness coach, I support the inclusion of animal-assisted treatment as an adjunctive strategy in the all-encompassing care of Alzheimer's patients. A higher quality of life, as well as a sense of joy and companionship that is genuinely irreplaceable, can be experienced by those living with this disease by acknowledging and utilising the healing power of animals.

Environmental Modifications for Cognitive Support

Chapter 4: Environmental Modifications for Cognitive Support

Introduction

As a physician and health and wellness coach, I have personally seen the effects that changes to the environment may have on people who have Alzheimer's disease. Alzheimer's is a multifaceted illness that impacts behaviour, emotional stability, memory, and cognitive function. We can help people with Alzheimer's disease live better lives and maintain their cognitive abilities by making certain changes to their physical surroundings.

Understanding the Role of the Environment

2.1 The Impact of Environment on Cognitive Function

Studies have demonstrated that the physical surroundings can have a major impact on cognitive performance. The lighting, noise level, and general design of the space can all help or hurt a person's ability to think clearly. Environmental adjustments are essential for preserving cognitive function and lowering confusion and agitation in Alzheimer's patients.

2.2 Creating a Dementia-Friendly Environment

An setting that is created with dementia patients' specific needs and difficulties in mind is called dementia-friendly. It is an environment that fosters self-reliance, security, and a feeling of familiarity. We can establish such an environment that promotes general well-being and cognitive function by putting particular tactics and adjustments into practise.

Strategies for Environmental Modifications

3.1 Lighting

Lighting is one of the most important factors of environmental alterations. By reducing glare and shadows, proper lighting enhances visual perception and lessens confusion. While natural light is ideal, plenty of artificial lighting should be available in situations when it isn't. Furthermore, by using contrasting hues in the space, people with Alzheimer's disease may find it easier to see essential regions and items.

3.2 Noise Reduction

For people with Alzheimer's, excessive noise can be overpowering and distracting. Setting up a peaceful space is crucial to supporting their cognitive abilities. This can be done by creating quiet spaces where people can go to relax and unwind, lowering background noise from appliances and devices, and utilising sound-absorbing materials to reduce echoes.

3.3 Color and Contrast

Effective use of colour and contrast can aid in the distinction between items and spaces for those suffering from Alzheimer's. High contrast colours can improve eye perception by drawing attention to specific items. A relaxing and tranquil atmosphere can also be produced by utilising colours that are familiar and elicit pleasant feelings and recollections.

3.4 Simplified Layout

People suffering from Alzheimer's disease may find complex and congested environments disorienting and puzzling. We can make the area for them easier to use and more intuitive by going with a more straightforward layout. Minimal furniture, clearly marked objects, and clear walkways can all aid in fostering independence and lowering uncertainty.

3.5 Safety Measures

Ensuring a secure atmosphere is crucial for effectively handling Alzheimer's disease. This entails removing trip hazards, fastening furniture, and utilising handrails and grab bars as safety measures. By adding locks and alarms to windows and doors, you can help keep people with dementia secure by preventing them from wandering.

Psychological and Emotional Well-being

4.1 Creating Familiarity

The process of making an environment dementia-friendly include adding objects and features that bring back happy memories. For those with Alzheimer's, sentimental items, intimate photos, and comforting smells can all help foster a sense of familiarity and familiarity.

4.2 Promoting Independence

In order to preserve cognitive function and uphold one's dignity, independence must be encouraged. Individuals suffering from Alzheimer's disease can preserve their sense of independence by setting up areas and offering cues that help with daily tasks. Incorporating assistive technologies that promote independence, labelling cabinets and drawers, and employing visual reminders are a few examples of how to do this.

4.3 Calming and Sensory Stimulation

Adding sensory components can soothe and calm people in addition to making the space comfortable and empowering. Calm environments can be produced with the help of soft music, comforting aromas, and tactile stimulation like textured surfaces or objects.

Conclusion

In summary, environmental changes are important for managing Alzheimer's disease. We can promote cognitive performance, lessen confusion and agitation, and enhance the general well-being of people with Alzheimer's by implementing targeted changes to the physical environment. All aspects of the environment, including lighting, layout, safety features, and psychological support, can be tailored to make a home dementia-friendly. By employing all-encompassing and holistic methods for managing Alzheimer's disease, we can offer people the assistance and attention they need as they progress toward optimal health.

Integrative Approaches and Personalized Plans

Throughout the years that I have worked as a medical doctor and a health and wellness coach, I have learned that every person is different, with different requirements and situations. This is particularly true with a disease as complex and incapacitating as Alzheimer's. Creating individualised plans that take into account each patient's goals, preferences, lifestyle, and medical history is crucial to delivering genuinely successful treatment.

In terms of controlling Alzheimer's Disease, there is no one-size-fits-all approach. A customised plan guarantees that the therapeutic strategy considers the unique requirements of the patient, giving them the ideal opportunity to enhance their quality of life and impede the disease's advancement.

Undertaking a thorough assessment is the first step towards creating a customised plan. A thorough medical history must be obtained, a physical examination must be performed, and the person's cognitive and functional abilities must be evaluated. Determining the most appropriate interventions requires knowledge of the individual's baseline health as well as the present condition of the disease.

To give a comprehensive approach to managing Alzheimer's disease, I collaborate closely with a group of specialists from several health and wellness domains. Practitioners of alternative therapy, psychologists, counsellors, and dietitians make up this team. We can address not just the physical symptoms but also the emotional, psychological, and spiritual facets of an individual's well-being by combining medical interventions with holistic techniques.

A key component of managing Alzheimer's disease is changing one's lifestyle. Studies have indicated that specific lifestyle factors may have a role in the onset and advancement of the disease. A bad diet,

Chapter 4: Customizable Plans for Alzheimer's Disease Management

Cognitive Stimulation Plan

It's important to comprehend the reasoning behind cognitive stimulation before getting into the particular exercises and methods. Cognitive skills including memory, reasoning, and thinking are all compromised by Alzheimer's disease, which affects the brain. By subjecting the brain to tasks that both test and stimulate its many processes, cognitive stimulation seeks to reverse this deterioration. Regular brain exercise can strengthen and create new neural connections, which will ultimately improve cognitive function.

Individualization is a crucial component of an effective plan for cognitive stimulation. Every person with Alzheimer's disease is different, and this includes their cognitive capacities as well as their preferences. As such, it is imperative that the workouts and activities be customised to the individual's unique requirements and interests. We can make sure they are engaged and get the most out of cognitive stimulation by doing this.

This subsection will provide an overview of different methods and exercises that can be included in a cognitive stimulation programme. It has been demonstrated that these techniques are beneficial for improving brain health and cognitive performance. I'll also offer advice on how to modify these exercises based on the person's specific stage of Alzheimer's.

1. Memory Activities:

One of the main objectives of cognitive stimulation is memory improvement. Depending on the ability of the person, memory exercises can be simple or difficult. Here are a few instances:

- Memory games: Engaging in memory games, like card matching or sequence recall, can improve brain function by practising information retention.

- Reminiscence therapy: Memorization-stirring activities like glancing at old photos or listening to well-known music can aid in promoting memory recall.

2. Cognitive Exercises:

The goal of cognitive exercises is to enhance a variety of cognitive functions, such as language, attention, problem-solving, and spatial awareness. Among the exercises that work well are:

- Crossword puzzles and word games: These exercises test one's ability to communicate and solve problems, which supports the preservation and improvement of cognitive capacities.

- Sudoku and crossword puzzles: By encouraging critical thinking and problem-solving abilities, these puzzles can improve cognitive function.

3. Social Engagement:

An essential component of cognitive stimulation is social interaction. Social interaction delivers emotional support in addition to brain stimulation. Among the social activities are:

- Group discussions: Getting people with Alzheimer's disease involved in group conversations can improve their cognitive function and give them a feeling of community.

- Volunteer work: Participating in volunteer work fosters social connection and a feeling of purpose, both of which are beneficial to cognitive health in general.

4. Physical Exercise:

Exercise is frequently disregarded while discussing cognitive stimulation. On the other hand, a number of studies have demonstrated that consistent physical exercise can improve cognitive performance. A few things to think about are:

- Walking: Walking quickly can increase blood flow to the brain, which makes it easier for the body to deliver the nutrients and oxygen needed for the best possible cognitive performance.

- Yoga: Yoga enhances mental clarity and relaxation in addition to increasing physical flexibility, all of which are beneficial to cognitive health.

5. Artistic Expression:

Creating things can activate different parts of the brain and improve mental functions. Consider engaging in the following artistic endeavours:

- Painting or drawing: Making art can help you express yourself and use your brain's visual-spatial abilities.

- Music therapy: Music can improve overall cognitive function, elicit strong emotional reactions, and increase memory recall.

It is significant to remember that the aforementioned activities are merely suggestions for creating a thorough schedule of cognitive stimulation; they are by no means exhaustive. Additionally, it is imperative that these activities be modified as the person advances through the various phases of Alzheimer's disease. Simpler, more structured activities may become necessary as the condition progresses because cognitive abilities may deteriorate.

Approaching cognitive stimulation also requires encouragement, adaptability, and patience. It is important to offer emotional support and confidence throughout the procedure, as individuals with Alzheimer's disease may occasionally exhibit resistance or dissatisfaction. Moreover, a regular regimen that includes cognitive stimulation might be quite beneficial. Maintaining a consistent schedule of stimulating activities is essential for reaping the greatest rewards.

Creating a strategy for cognitive stimulation is essential to controlling Alzheimer's disease, to sum up. People with Alzheimer's disease can enhance cognitive performance and advance brain health by involving their brains in activities that excite and test their many functions. Individuals can have improved cognitive capacities and a higher quality of life by implementing memory exercises, cognitive exercises, physical exercise, social involvement, and artistic expression. Never forget that every strategy needs to be customised for the specific needs, abilities, and stage of Alzheimer's disease of each person. Cognitive stimulation can play a crucial role in controlling Alzheimer's disease and enhancing general wellbeing if it is applied with persistence, encouragement, and patience.

Nutritional Plan for Brain Health

I've worked for years as a medical practitioner and health and wellness coach, and during that time I've learned how important nutrition is to brain function. Research has demonstrated that some eating patterns can lower the risk of cognitive decline and enhance general brain function when paired with other lifestyle changes. A nutritious diet that is well-balanced can help maintain brain function and possibly lower the risk of Alzheimer's disease.

Dietary Recommendations:

A balanced and diverse diet should be the top priority when creating a nutritional plan for brain health. The positive effects of the Mediterranean diet on the brain have been thoroughly explored. The majority of the foods in this eating pattern are plant-based and include fruits, vegetables, whole grains, legumes, and nuts. It also limits red meat and processed foods and incorporates fish, chicken, and dairy products in moderation. Healthy fats, such as the monounsaturated fats in olive oil, are abundant in the Mediterranean diet and have been linked to a lower incidence of cognitive decline.

The DASH (Dietary Approaches to Stop Hypertension) diet concepts can also be incorporated to support brain health. Consuming fruits, vegetables, whole grains, lean proteins, low-fat dairy products, and limiting sodium and saturated fat intake are all important components of the DASH diet. It has been demonstrated that this diet enhances cognitive performance in addition to lowering blood pressure.

Meal Planning Strategies:

A thoughtfully prepared meal serves as the cornerstone of a diet for brain health. Every meal should include a range of meals to guarantee that the brain is getting a continuous supply of nutrients. I advise my patients to eat a variety of whole grains, fruits, vegetables, lean meats, and healthy fats every day. The following meal planning techniques can promote mental wellness:

1. Focus on whole foods: Choose whole foods over processed ones because they are higher in vital nutrients and contain less harmful fats and added sugars. Refined grains should be avoided in favour of whole grains like quinoa, brown rice, and whole wheat bread.

2. Colorful fruits and vegetables: A rainbow of fruits and vegetables should be your goal because they offer an abundance of different antioxidants, vitamins, and minerals. Incorporate cruciferous veggies, such as broccoli and cauliflower, into your meals along with leafy greens, berries, tomatoes, and avocados.

3. Incorporate healthy fats: Eat foods high in avocados, nuts, seeds, and fatty fish (sardines, mackerel, and salmon) as well as other sources of good fats. Omega-3 fatty acids, which are present in these lipids, have been demonstrated to promote brain function.

4. Limit added sugars and unhealthy fats: Overindulgence in harmful fats and added sweets can be detrimental to brain function. Reduce your consumption of processed snacks, sugar-filled beverages, and foods high in trans and saturated fats.

Specific Nutrients for Cognitive Function:

A few key nutrients are essential for maintaining brain health and cognitive function. By making sure we are getting enough of these nutrients, we can enhance brain function in general and memory in particular. A diet plan for brain health should contain the following essential nutrients:

1. Omega-3 fatty acids: Omega-3 fatty acids are vital for brain function and can be found in walnuts, chia seeds, flaxseeds, and fatty fish. They support the structure of brain cells and have anti-inflammatory and anti-oxidant properties that can help prevent cognitive decline.

2. Antioxidants: Antioxidants aid in shielding the brain from harm brought on by free radicals. Incorporate antioxidant-rich meals like dark chocolate, berries, green tea, and vibrant fruits and vegetables.

3. B vitamins: B vitamins are essential for healthy brain function, especially vitamin B12. They are involved in the upkeep of nerve cells as well as the synthesis of neurotransmitters. Meat, fish, eggs, and dairy products are examples of animal items that are good sources of vitamin B12. For those on a plant-based diet, such as vegans or vegetarians, fortified foods or supplements could be required.

4. Vitamin D: Dementia risk and cognitive impairment have been related to vitamin D deficiency. To help your skin produce vitamin D from sunshine, spend time outside. You can also think about including foods high in vitamin D, such eggs, dairy products, and fatty fish.

5. Magnesium: Because it affects synaptic plasticity and neurotransmitter release, magnesium is necessary for proper brain function. Consume foods high in magnesium, such as leafy greens, legumes, nuts, and seeds.

6. Curcumin: The key ingredient in turmeric, curcumin, has been shown to possess antioxidant and anti-inflammatory qualities. Additionally, it might aid in removing the amyloid plaques that are a hallmark of Alzheimer's disease. Think about taking pills or incorporating turmeric into your diet.

In summary, maintaining a healthy brain function and possibly lowering the risk of cognitive decline require a well-designed nutritional regimen. One may make sure they are getting a well-balanced intake of nutrients that support brain health by adhering to dietary recommendations, such as the DASH and Mediterranean diets, and utilising meal planning tools. To optimise cognitive performance, don't forget to incorporate certain nutrients in your diet, such as antioxidants, B vitamins, vitamin D, magnesium, and curcumin. Speak with a certified dietician or healthcare provider to create a customised eating plan that meets your needs. You can boost overall wellbeing and nourish your brain with the right diet and lifestyle choices.

Physical Exercise and Fitness Plan

Numerous advantages of physical activity have been demonstrated for those suffering from Alzheimer's disease. Frequent exercise enhances cardiovascular health, circulation, and general physical fitness. It also lowers the chance of developing other chronic illnesses like diabetes and heart disease and helps maintain a healthy weight. In fact, neuroplasticity—the brain's capacity to change and create new connections—has been discovered to be enhanced by exercise. This is particularly significant for those who have Alzheimer's disease.

It can be difficult for people with Alzheimer's disease to include physical activity into their daily schedule, especially as the condition worsens. Nonetheless, different exercise regimens are appropriate for various disease stages. Walking, swimming, and dancing are examples of effective early activities, when people are still able to engage in more sophisticated activities. These pursuits encourage social connection and mental stimulation in addition to physical activity.

People may need more specialised exercises that take into consideration their unique strengths and limits as the condition worsens. Exercises that target balance, coordination, and strength training can assist to increase mobility and lower the risk of falls in people with Alzheimer's disease who are in the intermediate stages of the disease. Yoga, tai chi, and resistance training with small weights or resistance bands are a few examples of these workouts.

Even in the later stages of Alzheimer's disease, when a person may have diminished cognitive function and mobility, basic movement exercises and mild stretching can be helpful. You can perform these exercises while seated or with a caregiver's help. Seated yoga, chair aerobics, and gentle stretching are a few examples. Physical and mental health can benefit from even brief bursts of movement and activity.

It takes great thought and preparation to include physical activity in an Alzheimer's disease patient's daily routine. It is critical to consider the person's safety, preferences, and talents. The following are some methods for adding exercise to regular schedules:

1. Start with a visit to the doctor: It is crucial to speak with a healthcare provider before beginning any physical activity programme, ideally one who is knowledgeable in Alzheimer's disease. They are able to evaluate the person's general health and offer suggestions for appropriate workout regimens.

2. Set realistic goals: Setting attainable goals that consider each person's strengths and weaknesses is crucial. Set modest, attainable initial targets and work your way up to longer, more intense workouts over time.

3. Make it enjoyable: Select pursuits that are important and enjoyable for the person. Take up mentally stimulating and joyful hobbies like dancing, gardening, or music-making. When it is feasible, include social interaction since this can further amplify the advantages of physical activity.

4. Create a routine: Create a regular physical activity regimen and integrate it into the person's everyday routine. This can guarantee that they incorporate exercise into their daily routine and help them form a habit of doing so.

5. Modify and adapt: It can be required to adjust and modify workouts as the disease worsens in order to account for changes in cognitive and physical ability. This could entail making motions simpler, lowering the level of difficulty or duration of the workouts, or offering more help and support.

6. Monitor progress: Observe the person's development and modify the workout regimen as necessary. Make sure the workouts are safe but also difficult by periodically evaluating their skills and modifying the programme as needed.

7. Involve caregivers and support networks: enlist the assistance of caregivers and other people in the person's support system. They can

support and encourage the person to engage in physical activity, help during workouts, and watch out for their safety.

In conclusion, adding exercise to a person's regular routine can help them much both mentally and physically, especially if they have Alzheimer's disease. Exercise plays a critical role in managing Alzheimer's Disease, from enhancing neuroplasticity and general brain health to enhancing cardiovascular health and mobility. People with Alzheimer's Disease can still enjoy active, satisfying lives by designing a personalised fitness programme that takes into consideration their talents and limits and by including physical activity into their daily routines. With the use of this framework, I intend to help people with Alzheimer's disease and their caregivers create a physical activity and fitness plan that will improve their overall quality of life and provide them direction and support.

Sleep Hygiene and Restful Sleep Plan

Sleep Hygiene: The Foundation of Restful Sleep

Developing a healthy sleep hygiene regimen is essential to getting a decent night's sleep. The term "sleep hygiene" describes a collection of actions and habits that support increased quantities and quality of sleep. People suffering from Alzheimer's disease can enhance their general health and quality of sleep by adhering to these tips.

1. Establish a Consistent Bedtime Routine: The body's internal clock can be regulated by following a regular nighttime regimen. This regimen ought to consist of things like having a warm bath, relaxing with exercises, reading light literature, or listening to calming music. It is easier to fall asleep and stay asleep through the night when you stick to a regular schedule because your brain interprets these cues as signals to go to sleep.

2. Create a Sleep-Friendly Environment: Our sleeping environment has a big influence on how well we sleep. Ensure that the bedroom is dark, quiet, and at a temperature that suits you. To reduce visual disturbances, use blackout curtains or eye masks; to reduce noise, use white noise machines or earplugs. Furthermore, purchasing cosy pillows and mattresses can greatly enhance the comfort of sleep.

3. Limit Stimulants and Avoid Heavy Meals Before Bed: It is well known that stimulants like caffeine and nicotine can disrupt sleep. Avoiding these substances is advised, especially in the afternoon and evening. In a similar vein, eating large meals right before bed can induce indigestion and discomfort, which makes it harder to fall asleep. If need be, choose light, easily digested foods instead.

4. Avoid Long Naps During the Day: Long daytime naps can throw off the sleep-wake cycle, even though short power naps might be helpful for certain people. Napping should be restricted to no more than 20 to 30 minutes, ideally in the morning.

5. Regular Physical Activity: Regular daytime exercise has been demonstrated to enhance the quality of sleep. But it's crucial to schedule physical activity properly; avoid doing intense workouts just before bed since this can make you more alert and make it harder to fall asleep. Walking and other gentle workouts like yoga can help to encourage sound sleep.

Managing Sleep Disturbances in Alzheimer's Disease

Because of the nature of the condition, people with Alzheimer's may still have sleep problems even if they adhere to the aforementioned sleep hygiene guidelines. Nighttime wandering, trouble falling asleep, frequent awakenings, and excessive daytime tiredness are a few examples of these disruptions. Here are some methods to deal with these typical Alzheimer's disease sleep problems:

1. Addressing Nighttime Wandering: One common sign of Alzheimer's disease is nighttime roaming, which can be dangerous. Make sure the residence is safe with locks on the windows and doors to help lessen this. To lessen restlessness at night, create a regular bedtime routine and make an effort to keep the individual active during the day. During nocturnal wanderings, bright nightlights in corridors and bathrooms can help prevent falls.

2. Promoting Relaxation Techniques: Using relaxation techniques can be beneficial for people who have trouble falling asleep. Deep breathing techniques, progressive muscular relaxation, meditation, and guided imagery are a few examples of this. These methods support a more relaxed state that is favourable for sleeping by calming the body and mind.

3. Managing Frequent Awakenings: It can be difficult to deal with frequent awakenings, but there are techniques that can be useful. Make sure the bedroom is first comfy and devoid of distractions that could keep you from sleeping. In order to prevent upsetting the person further if they wake up in the middle of the night, reassure them and

speak in a kind, calming tone. Steer clear of strong lighting and distracting activities.

4. Addressing Excessive Daytime Sleepiness: A person's everyday functioning and quality of life may be negatively impacted by excessive daytime sleepiness. To make sure the person has adequate exposure to natural light during the day, it's critical to keep a regular sleep-wake pattern. Reducing daytime sleepiness can also be achieved by participating in activities that stimulate the body and mind during the day.

Recall that every person with Alzheimer's disease is different, and this includes the sleep difficulties they experience. For individualised advice and suggestions, speaking with a medical expert who specialises in dementia care or sleep difficulties may be beneficial.

For those suffering from Alzheimer's disease, creating a customised sleep hygiene routine and peaceful sleep schedule calls for persistence, comprehension, and continuous adjustment. People with Alzheimer's can experience better sleep quality and general well-being by putting these ideas into practise and prioritising sleep.

Stress Management and Relaxation Techniques

As a physician and health and wellness coach, I have personally witnessed the advantages of adding stress reduction and relaxation methods to my patients' treatment regimens for Alzheimer's disease. These methods support a feeling of general well-being, boost mood, increase cognitive performance, and lower stress levels.

I'll give you a step-by-step tutorial in this subchapter on creating a stress-reduction and relaxation programme that is especially catered to the needs of people with Alzheimer's disease. Every phase will concentrate on a distinct method, such as progressive muscle relaxation, guided visualisation, and deep breathing, all of which have been studied and found to be beneficial in lowering stress levels.

Deep Breathing

Anywhere, at any time, deep breathing is a straightforward, yet effective method that may be performed. It entails inhaling deeply and slowly via the nose, holding the breath for a little while, and then slowly releasing the breath through the mouth. In addition to triggering the body's relaxation response, deep breathing helps lessen the physical signs of stress, such as stiff muscles and a fast heartbeat.

Choose a peaceful, cosy spot to sit or lie down to begin practising deep breathing. Shut your eyes and concentrate on your breathing for a brief while. Breathe in deeply and slowly through your nose while you count to four. After holding your breath for four counts, gently release it through your mouth while continuing to count to four. For a few minutes, repeat this exercise while concentrating only on your breathing and letting go of any other distracting ideas or concerns.

Progressive Muscle Relaxation

A method called progressive muscle relaxation entails methodically tensing and relaxing various bodily muscle groups. This method aids in promoting relaxation, easing tense muscles, and lowering anxiety. It is especially helpful for people with Alzheimer's disease since it helps relieve agitation and encourage serenity.

The first step in practising progressive muscle relaxation is to settle into a comfortable position and inhale deeply several times. Starting with your toes, curl them tightly and hold them for a little while before letting go of the tension and allowing your toes to fully relax. Tensing and relaxing each muscle area, go to your calves, thighs, belly, chest, arms, hands, and lastly your face. Consider the sensations of tension and relaxation as you work through each muscle group, and make an effort to release all of the stress you may be carrying within.

Guided Imagery

Using the power of the imagination, guided imagery is a technique that helps people relax and cope with stress. It entails visualising serene and tranquil settings, such a beach or a forest, and losing yourself entirely in the sensory aspects of these visions. By diverting the mind from nervous ideas and concerns, guided imagery can promote inner calm and serenity.

To engage in guided visualisation exercises, locate a peaceful, cosy spot to sit or recline. To calm your body and mind, close your eyes and take several deep breaths. Next, picture yourself in a calm and serene setting of your choosing. Imagine all of the specifics of this place, including the hues, noises, and scents. Envision yourself completely engrossed in this landscape, experiencing a wave of serenity and tranquilly. For as long as you like, spend some time in this imagined location, relishing the tranquil feelings and releasing any tension or stress.

Regular Practice and Implementation

It's critical to practise these stress-reduction and relaxation techniques on a regular basis and integrate them into your daily routine in order to fully benefit from them. Organize your time so that you may practise progressive muscle relaxation, guided imagery, or deep breathing at a set time every day, or add these techniques to your current self-care regimen. Since consistency is essential, resolve to put your mental health first and include these methods into your daily routine.

It's critical to identify and deal with any underlying sources of stress in your life in addition to these strategies. This could entail adopting constructive coping mechanisms, asking for help from family members or a therapist, and changing one's lifestyle as needed. It's important to keep in mind that self-care should come first and that managing your stress and encouraging relaxation are critical to your general wellbeing.

You may greatly enhance your emotional health and general quality of life by adopting these stress-reduction and relaxation strategies into your daily routine and taking care of the underlying causes of stress in your life. Always remember to practise self-compassion and grant yourself permission to put your own well-being first. These methods will come naturally to you with time and practise, and you'll see the great effects they can have on your life.

In summary, a thorough management strategy for Alzheimer's disease must include stress reduction and relaxation approaches. You can lower stress, improve cognitive performance, and foster emotional well-being by making deep breathing, progressive muscle relaxation, and guided visualisation a regular part of your routine. Don't forget to put these strategies into daily practise and deal with any underlying stressors in your life. You can improve your quality of life and learn the art of stress management with perseverance and devotion.

Social Engagement and Support Network Plan

As I explore the role that social networks and engagement play in managing Alzheimer's disease, I can't help but think of all the people I have seen throughout my medical career. I have seen firsthand how social ties can improve the quality of life for individuals living with Alzheimer's disease in addition to helping to manage the disease's symptoms.

Humans are social animals with profound innate social interaction needs. Because we are social beings, the relationships we have with other people have a profound impact on our mental and emotional well-being. Building social ties is much more important for those who have Alzheimer's disease. Research indicates that upholding an engaged social circle can promote cognitive abilities, postpone cognitive deterioration, and augment the general standard of living for individuals afflicted with Alzheimer's Disease. This is the reason I stress the significance of creating a thorough plan for social engagement and support networks as part of your management approach for Alzheimer's disease.

This subchapter will walk you through the process of developing a customised strategy that includes methods for establishing and sustaining relationships, making social connections, and gaining access to resources for help. Recall that there is no one-size-fits-all strategy with this plan. Using these tactics requires taking into account the patient's particular needs, preferences, and disease stage.

Assessing Social Needs and Preferences

Assembling your Social Engagement and Support Network Plan begins with determining the social needs and preferences of the Alzheimer's patient. Spend some time in frank and open communication with your loved one to learn about their preferences for social engagement, including the kinds of activities they like to do and the individuals who make them feel most at ease. Keep in mind that this is a cooperative process, and giving the Alzheimer's patient a voice in decisions empowers them and fosters a sense of independence.

Identifying Social Activities

After you have a firm grasp on the person's preferences and social demands, you should find social activities that suit their interests. The goal is to partake in activities that enhance emotional health, foster social contact, and boost cognitive performance. Think about getting involved in community activities, taking part in Alzheimer's support groups in your area, or pursuing interests and hobbies that encourage social interaction. Family and friends can have a big impact on an individual's feeling of belonging and mental health, so encourage them to join part.

Cultivating Relationships

For those suffering from Alzheimer's disease, preserving relationships is crucial since it offers a sense of familiarity, comfort, and emotional support. Promote consistent communication with loved ones, close companions, and well-known individuals in the neighbourhood. Arrange meetings, events, and visits in a way that best suits the person's preferences and cognitive skills. Activities might need to be modified to make sure everyone can participate and find them entertaining and doable.

Building a Support Network

It's important to keep up current relationships and establish a support system of people who are aware of the difficulties associated with having Alzheimer's disease. Online and in-person support groups can offer priceless guidance, emotional support, and a feeling of community. Through sharing and learning from one another's experiences, these groups enable people to create a supportive environment, which is crucial for navigating the intricacies of Alzheimer's disease. Consult healthcare experts who specialise in managing Alzheimer's disease, such as social workers, psychologists, and counsellors. These professionals can offer priceless information and tools that can improve your network of support in general.

Enhancing Communication Strategies

As Alzheimer's disease worsens, it can be harder to communicate. Effective communication techniques, however, can lessen irritation for the person with Alzheimer's Disease and their loved ones while also preserving meaningful ties. Encourage family members and caregivers to use non-verbal indicators, visual aids, and straightforward language when communicating with one another. Additionally, inform others in their immediate vicinity of the increasing nature of Alzheimer's disease, assisting them in comprehending the alterations in communication skills and figuring out how to modify their interactions appropriately.

Addressing Safety Concerns

It's important to deal with safety concerns early on when participating in social activities. Enforcing safety precautions, like identity wristbands or tags bearing emergency contact details, can reduce anxieties and guarantee that the person suffering from Alzheimer's Disease can join in social activities without risk. Make sure that their living space is safe and clear of any threats that could endanger their health as well.

Integrating Technology into Social Engagement

In the current digital era, there are many tools and services available thanks to technology that can help people with Alzheimer's Disease participate in social activities. To facilitate virtual relationships with family and friends who might not be there in person, think about using video chat systems. Additionally, there are instruments for reminiscence therapy and digital memory aides that help improve memory recall and cognitive performance.

Evolving the Social Engagement and Support Network Plan

Since Alzheimer's is a degenerative disorder, the Social Engagement and Support Network Plan needs to be reviewed and updated on a regular basis. Evaluate the person's social requirements and preferences on a regular basis, and modify support systems and activities as necessary. To make sure the plan is thorough and current, keep up with new findings, treatments, and services available to people with Alzheimer's disease.

Through adherence to these guidelines and the execution of a meticulously designed Social Engagement and Support Network Plan, people diagnosed with Alzheimer's Disease can sustain a vibrant social life, cultivate significant connections, and obtain the assistance required to effectively manage the disease's obstacles. Recall that every person's experience with Alzheimer's disease is different, and that's why it's so important to treat them with respect and understanding of their specific requirements and preferences. By working together, we can revolutionise the way Alzheimer's disease is treated and enable individuals who are impacted to lead meaningful, fulfilling lives with dignity.

Self-Care and Coping Strategies

The foundation of self-care is self-compassion, which enables us to be kind and understanding to ourselves. It can be extremely difficult to live with Alzheimer's disease for both the person who has been diagnosed and their loved ones. It is important to keep in mind that it is acceptable to experience frustration, fear, or even rage occasionally. Being able to recognise and deal with these feelings is the first step in developing self-compassion.

Mindfulness is one method that can help develop self-compassion. Intentionally focusing on the current moment while avoiding passing judgement is known as mindfulness. By engaging in mindfulness practises, we open up a space inside of ourselves to notice our feelings and thoughts without becoming caught up in them. We can better comprehend our experiences and respond to them with self-compassion if we can cultivate this non-judgmental awareness.

Reducing stress is another effective coping mechanism. It has been demonstrated that prolonged stress has a detrimental effect on one's physical and mental well-being, making Alzheimer's disease patients' struggles more severe. In my capacity as a physician and health and wellness coach, I have witnessed firsthand the life-changing potential of stress-reduction strategies for my patients.

Deep breathing exercises are one approach that has shown promise in reducing stress. Breathing slowly and deeply stimulates the parasympathetic nerve system of the body, hence reducing the stress reaction. You may effectively lower your stress levels by helping your body to go into a relaxation response by setting aside a little amount of time each day to concentrate on your breathing.

I advise doing progressive muscular relaxation in addition to deep breathing techniques. To remove built-up stress, this technique entails methodically tensing and then relaxing certain muscle groups.

Focusing on each muscle group and actively releasing tension might help you tell your body when it's okay to let go.

Getting regular exercise is just another effective way to reduce stress. It has been demonstrated that exercise releases endorphins, which are organic mood boosters. In addition, exercise gives us a feeling of empowerment and success that helps us deal with the difficulties associated with Alzheimer's disease.

Keep in mind that every person has unique strengths and limitations, and that you should always seek medical advice before starting a new fitness programme. It's advisable to select a hobby or pastime that complements your physical capabilities and brings you satisfaction. Regular activity, whether it be swimming, walking, or even chair workouts, can significantly improve your general health.

For the management of Alzheimer's disease, developing emotional resilience is just as important as practising self-compassion and reducing stress. The term "emotional resilience" describes the capacity to adjust and overcome hardship. Even though Alzheimer's disease presents many difficulties, you can deal with its unpredictability more easily if you have emotional resilience.

Cognitive restructuring is one method that supports emotional resilience. Reframing negative thought patterns in a more empowering and positive way is the process of cognitive restructuring. You can develop emotional fortitude and resilience by making the deliberate decision to see setbacks as chances for development and education.

Including fun things in your daily schedule might also help you become more emotionally resilient. Taking up hobbies or following passions can give you a sense of fulfilment and purpose that improves your emotional health. Discovering hobbies that you enjoy, whether it's painting, gardening, or learning to play an instrument, can be a very effective coping strategy.

Creating a network of support can also significantly improve emotional resilience. Making connections with people who are experiencing similar things to you can help you feel like you belong and create a space where you can share and learn. Finding online communities or taking part in support groups can provide a lot of understanding and support.

In summary, the development of coping mechanisms and self-care is essential to managing Alzheimer's disease. Adopting self-compassion, stress management strategies, and emotional resilience can help you manage the difficulties of Alzheimer's Disease and improve your general well-being. Never forget that it's acceptable to prioritise your own health and to seek for assistance. Together, we can design a comprehensive management plan for Alzheimer's disease that is specific to your needs and situation.

Integrating Medical and Holistic Approaches

Alzheimer's disease is a complicated illness that impacts a person's general wellbeing in addition to their cognitive functioning. As a physician and health and wellness coach, I have seen firsthand the drawbacks of treating a sickness only with pharmaceuticals.

Medical interventions, such as medication, can assist manage certain symptoms and slow down the illness's progression, but they frequently are not sufficient to meet the needs of people with Alzheimer's disease on a holistic level. This is the point at which using holistic methods becomes essential.

The goal of holistic medicine is to treat the patient as a whole, mind, body, and spirit. It acknowledges that achieving optimal health requires striking a balance between one's physical and mental well-being, emotional stability, and social ties, among other areas of one's life. The integration of medical and holistic treatments can yield a more comprehensive and individualised approach to the therapy of Alzheimer's disease.

Forming a team of specialists from various health and wellness domains is the first step towards combining medical and holistic treatments. Together, the members of this team will create a personalised treatment plan for the patient that takes into consideration their unique requirements and preferences.

Physicians, naturopaths, dietitians, psychologists, therapists, and other healthcare practitioners with a focus on holistic health may make up the team. They will work together to provide a multifaceted approach to Alzheimer's disease management.

Lifestyle changes are one of the main elements of the integrated care plan. Studies have indicated that specific lifestyle choices can have a major effect on cognitive function and brain health. Incorporating lifestyle changes like consistent exercise, a healthy diet, stress reduction methods, and restful sleep can improve general health and possibly halt the advancement of some diseases.

Particularly exercise has been demonstrated to improve brain health. Walking and swimming are examples of aerobic exercises that have been shown to enhance cognitive function and lower the risk of Alzheimer's disease. Conversely, resistance exercise can lessen the chance of accidents and falls by enhancing muscle strength and balance.

A balanced diet is also essential for preserving brain function. A diet high in omega-3 fatty acids, low in processed carbohydrates and saturated fats, and high in antioxidants has been found to aid prevent cognitive deterioration. A customised meal plan can be created in collaboration with a nutritionist to address the unique dietary requirements of those living with Alzheimer's disease.

It's crucial to remember that each person may experience different effects from lifestyle changes. As a result, routine monitoring and assessment should be carried out to determine their efficacy and make any required modifications to the care plan.

The integrated treatment plan must also include counselling and psychology-related techniques in addition to lifestyle adjustments. Alzheimer's disease impacts not just the patient but also caretakers and family members. It may make you feel depressed, irritated, and powerless. We can assist individuals and their families in overcoming the emotional and psychological obstacles associated with the illness by offering counselling and psychological support.

Several complementary and alternative methods of self-care might be included in the integrated care plan. Acupuncture, aromatherapy, massage therapy, and mindfulness exercises are a few possible techniques. Although there isn't much scientific proof to back them up, they have been shown to promote physical and emotional relaxation, lessen tension and anxiety, and enhance general wellbeing.

Alzheimer's patients may also benefit from self-help strategies including brain games, cognitive training programmes, and memory aides. These methods can help improve everyday functioning, memory retention, and cognitive performance.

Ultimately, coping mechanisms are essential to managing Alzheimer's disease. It might be difficult to accept the diagnosis and come to terms with the changes brought on by the illness. We can better assist people and their families in navigating the journey with Alzheimer's Disease by offering coping mechanisms including support groups, respite care, and educational opportunities.

Conclusively, the integration of medical and holistic treatments is necessary for the comprehensive care of Alzheimer's disease. The greatest aspects of both worlds can be combined to provide people a customised care plan that takes into account their unique requirements and preferences. By implementing lifestyle adjustments, counselling and psychology-related methods, alternative and complementary forms of self-care, self-help approaches, and coping mechanisms, we can enable patients and their families to take charge of their health and improve their general living conditions. By working together, we can design a comprehensive management plan for Alzheimer's disease.

Chapter 5: Living Well With Alzheimer's Disease

Finding Meaning and Purpose

Having worked closely with people coping with Alzheimer's disease for many years in my medical practise, I have learned that receiving the diagnosis itself may be stressful and depressing for both the patient and their loved ones. Finding meaning and purpose in life becomes even more important during these trying times. Many people have feelings of pessimism and despair after receiving an Alzheimer's diagnosis, which can lower their general level of wellbeing. But I really think that accepting meaning and purpose can change what it's like to have Alzheimer's, enabling people to live happy, full lives in spite of the inevitable obstacles that will inevitably arise.

So, in the face of Alzheimer's disease, what does it mean to find meaning and purpose? It starts with a self-discovery trip, during which people consider their values, beliefs, and the things that are most important to them. Through self-reflection, people can discover what gives their lives meaning and happiness despite the limitations caused by their illness. Understanding that one's life is a tapestry of experiences, relationships, and aspirations that are still unexplored is a necessary step in the process of finding meaning and purpose.

I frequently urge people to partake in activities that are in line with their passions and personal beliefs in order to support this discovery. This could be engaging in creative pursuits, volunteering for issues near and dear to their hearts, engaging in hobbies, or developing a stronger spiritual connection. In addition to providing happiness and contentment, these kinds of activities enhance mental and emotional health, build resilience, and help people deal with the difficulties associated with Alzheimer's disease.

Despite the restrictions of Alzheimer's, I have seen innumerable examples of people finding new ways to express themselves and find meaning and purpose. For instance, I remember a patient named Sarah who painted and found great joy and fulfilment, even though her illness was getting worse. She was able to express herself again and became an inspiration to other members of the Alzheimer's community because to art therapy. It made me think about how important it is to pursue passion and creative endeavours in order to develop a feeling of meaning and purpose in life.

While finding joy and fulfilment in one's activities is important, making meaningful goals can further strengthen one's feeling of purpose during one's Alzheimer's journey. Simple objectives like preserving one's bodily and mental health, developing deep relationships with loved ones, or making a lasting impression by advocating for causes and increasing public awareness of Alzheimer's disease might be included in this list. By pursuing these objectives, people get a feeling of purpose and direction that frequently exceeds their own expectations and prevents them from being defined only by their diagnosis.

It is imperative to recognise, nevertheless, that each person's journey toward discovering meaning and purpose within the framework of Alzheimer's disease is distinct. What gives one individual happiness and contentment could not have the same effect on another. Therefore, it's critical to approach this process of self-discovery with empathy and an open mind, enabling people to choose their own pathways and identify the things that give their lives meaning and purpose. In our capacity as healthcare professionals, we may encourage this investigation by providing direction, materials, and links to organisations or support groups that address the various interests and goals of individuals with Alzheimer's.

To sum up, the process of discovering meaning and purpose within the framework of Alzheimer's disease is an intensely personal and transforming experience. People who accept this part of who we are as human beings can face the obstacles posed by the illness with fortitude, optimism, and a feeling of purpose. People can learn that their lives are defined by the tales they tell, the connections they make, and the legacy they leave behind rather than only by their diagnosis by reflecting on themselves, doing joyful and fulfilling activities, and making significant goals. As medical professionals and caregivers, we have the honour of accompanying people on this journey and giving them the tools they need to develop a sense of purpose and meaning that goes beyond the limitations of Alzheimer's disease.

Enhancing Communication and Relationships

Case Study

Let me start by giving a compelling case study that highlights the significance of meaningful relationships and good communication in the setting of Alzheimer's disease. Introducing Mr. Robert, a 68-year-old man who was given an early-stage Alzheimer's diagnosis the previous year. As the principal caregiver for Mr. Robert, Mrs. Evelyn has observed notable shifts in his demeanour and communication skills.

Mr. Robert and his wife's communication grew more difficult and fragmented after he was initially diagnosed. He had trouble expressing himself, frequently mispronounced the names and faces of close relatives, and grew increasingly reclusive and aloof. Their relationship, which had previously been lively and affectionate, was now clouded by misunderstanding and frustration.

Upon observing Mrs. Evelyn's sorrow, I realised how important it was to step in and offer advice on improving communication and preserving a meaningful relationship despite the difficulties presented by Alzheimer's disease. We set out on a journey together to apply powerful communication tools, develop empathy, and discover methods to promote connection.

Effective Communication Techniques:

Adapting to the changes in a person's cognitive capacities and communication skills is crucial when it comes to improving communication in the context of Alzheimer's disease. It's critical to keep a courteous and upbeat attitude while being understanding, patient, and sympathetic.

1. Simplify language and use visual cues: As Alzheimer's disease worsens, people may find it harder to understand complicated concepts

or keep up with long conversations. When combined with visual aids like diagrams, charts, or gestures, short, to-the-point statements can assist close the gap in communication and improve comprehension.

2. Encourage non-verbal communication: Nonverbal cues can be very helpful in promoting comprehension and connection when verbal communication becomes more difficult. Promoting the use of gestures, expressions on the face, and body language can help successfully communicate feelings and wants.

3. Allow time for processing: It is crucial to keep in mind that people suffering from Alzheimer's disease could require more time to comprehend and react to stimuli. Allowing them enough time to collect their thoughts and reply at their own pace can help reduce annoyance and encourage productive dialogue.

Empathy-Building Strategies:

Developing empathy is crucial for establishing and preserving meaningful interactions with those who have Alzheimer's disease. It entails being aware of and sympathetic to their feelings, viewpoints, and experiences.

1. Active listening: Spend some time acknowledging and actively listening to the other person's feelings. Be really interested in what they have to say; don't cut them off or ignore their opinions. You may foster an atmosphere of safety and trust where candid conversation is encouraged by exhibiting empathy and acknowledging their feelings.

2. Validate their reality: People with Alzheimer's disease may get confused, lose their memories, or perceive time and events distortedly. Rather than criticising or refuting their experiences, it is imperative to meet them where they are and validate their reality. By doing this, unneeded stress can be avoided and comfort is encouraged.

3. Practice patience and compassion: People who suffer from Alzheimer's disease can display demanding or hard-to-understand behaviours. It is important to treat the problem with tolerance and compassion in such cases. Take a step back and try to comprehend the

underlying emotions that might be causing such conduct, rather than reacting with annoyance or fury.

Fostering Connection with Loved Ones:

People with Alzheimer's Disease can live far better lives if they continue to have meaningful interactions with their loved ones. It engenders happiness, security, and a sense of belonging. The following are some methods to promote connection:

1. Engaging in familiar activities: Promote engagement with former interests of the person suffering from Alzheimer's disease. Taking part in well-known pastimes, enjoying favourite music, or flipping through old photo albums can all aid in bringing back pleasant memories and feelings.

2. Creating a structured daily routine: A feeling of stability and predictability can be achieved by establishing a regular daily schedule. To create a cosy and familiar atmosphere, make sure that events like meals, excursions, and free time are planned in an orderly fashion.

3. Incorporating meaningful social interactions: Encourage the person to engage in regular social interactions with friends, family, and other important people in their life. Keeping in touch with loved ones via phone conversations, in-person visits, or video chats gives one a sense of community and emotional support.

Conclusion:

A key component of good caregiving and management is fostering meaningful relationships and improving communication despite the limitations presented by Alzheimer's disease. People with Alzheimer's Disease can live in a caring and supportive environment if we use good communication strategies, develop empathy, and make connections. Recall that every individual's experience is distinct, and managing the intricacies of Alzheimer's Disease calls for tolerance, comprehension, and flexibility.

Navigating Changes and Adapting to New Realities

One of the most upsetting parts of Alzheimer's disease is probably cognitive deterioration. Memory loss, disorientation, and trouble making decisions and solving problems get worse as the illness worsens. Although adjusting to these changes can be difficult, it's important to keep in mind that there are coping mechanisms available. Cognitive stimulation is one such tactic. Playing memory games, solving puzzles, and reading are examples of mentally taxing activities that can help prevent cognitive decline and enhance general brain function. Furthermore, maintaining social interactions and relationships with loved ones can offer cognitive and emotional support, making it easier for people with Alzheimer's disease to adjust to their changing abilities.

Another area that may require considerable adjustments is daily routines. Alzheimer's disease can cause routines to be upset and even simple tasks to become difficult. Setting a disciplined daily routine with attainable objectives is crucial for managing this. Activities can be made more approachable and feelings of overwhelm can be decreased by breaking them down into smaller, more manageable steps. It's also critical to give each activity adequate time, since rushing can exacerbate frustration and prevent a task from being completed successfully. Reminders and visual cues, such calendars and sticky notes, can be used to help people with Alzheimer's recall appointments and critical chores, giving them a sense of stability and order.

When handling the changes brought about by Alzheimer's Disease, flexibility and adaptation are essential. Adopting a mindset that recognises the situation's flexibility and permits adjustments as needed is crucial. This adaptability extends to the impacted person as well as to their support network and carers. Understanding that there may be new difficulties every day and lowering expectations appropriately can reduce stress and avert disappointment or frustration. It's also critical to ask for help and support when you need it, whether from medical professionals, support groups, or programmes for temporary relief from care. Establishing a solid support system can offer priceless direction, compassion, and understanding during this trying time.

A person's Alzheimer's care plan may also include a variety of additional tactics in addition to these strategies. Including complementary therapies like aromatherapy, music therapy, and pet therapy can stimulate the senses, encourage rest, and create a peaceful, well-being-inducing environment. These methods have demonstrated encouraging outcomes in lowering agitation, anxiety, and behavioural symptoms that are frequently connected to Alzheimer's disease.

The influence that adjusting to new circumstances and navigating changes presents in the setting of Alzheimer's Disease on caregivers is a topic that is frequently disregarded. It is impossible to overstate the mental, emotional, and physical toll that caring for a loved one with Alzheimer's takes. Caregivers' ability to offer care is greatly impacted by their general well-being, thus it is imperative that they prioritise self-care and get support. Maintaining caregiver health and avoiding burnout requires taking breaks, engaging in stress-reduction activities, and requesting respite care. Making connections with caregiver-specific therapy sessions or support groups can also offer a much-needed outlet for exchanging experiences, obtaining knowledge, and getting emotional support.

In addition, it's critical to recognise the emotional journey that comes with Alzheimer's. Alzheimer's patients and their loved ones may find it emotionally difficult to accept the diagnosis and the changes it brings about. Navigating the complicated emotions that surface might be greatly aided by attending counselling or therapy. A safe place to vent sadness, rage, and frustration can be found in therapy, and coping mechanisms for properly controlling these emotions can also be learned.

In summary, adjusting to new circumstances and navigating changes in the context of Alzheimer's disease necessitates a comprehensive strategy that includes cognitive stimulation, scheduling daily activities, embracing flexibility, putting complementary techniques into practise, and placing a high priority on the well-being of caregivers. Alzheimer's patients and their carers can develop a stronger sense of resilience, control, and well-being as they face future problems by implementing these methods into their management plans. Recall that you are not alone on this difficult road. You can find a method to deal with these changes and adjust to the new reality of Alzheimer's Disease with the right assistance and commitment.

Finding Joy in Everyday Moments

Essentially, mindfulness entails being totally aware of one's thoughts, feelings, and experiences while also being present in the moment. It promotes observation without passing judgement, which fosters acceptance and comprehension. When mindfulness is used to manage Alzheimer's disease, it can support emotional well-being, reduce stress, and improve quality of life for both patients and caregivers.

Mindfulness meditation is a particularly useful approach that entails focusing on the breath and nonjudgmentally noticing any thoughts or feelings that come. Depending on personal preferences and capacity, this practise can be continued for longer periods of time each day or shortened to as little as five minutes. Through the daily practise of mindfulness meditation, people can increase their ability to manage the difficulties associated with Alzheimer's disease in a calm and resilient manner.

Gratitude exercises are another helpful technique for discovering delight in the little things in life. Recognizing and enjoying life's blessings, no matter how minor or unimportant, is the essence of gratitude. Regular acts of thankfulness seem to have a good impact on mental health, general well-being, and outlook development, according to research.

I advise keeping a thankfulness notebook as a way to practise gratitude on a regular basis. Spend a few minutes every day listing three things for which you are thankful. These can be small pleasures like the beauty of nature, a warm cup of tea, or a kind act from a loved one. Through deliberate attention to these positive elements, people can change their perspective and adopt a happier, more appreciative attitude.

It's critical to learn methods for savouring happy memories in addition to mindfulness and gratitude exercises. Moments of happiness that might otherwise go unrecognised or underappreciated may be associated with Alzheimer's disease. Through purposeful appreciation of these times, people can improve their general state of wellbeing and find comfort in the face of difficulties.

A useful method for appreciating good things in life is "The Three S's." Using this method entails paying attention to the feelings, relishing the moment, and committing it to memory for future use. In the event that a patient receives a consoling hug from a loved one, for instance, they might consciously choose to remember the physical experience, relish the warmth and affection of that instant, and dedicate a time to fully appreciate the physical sensation.

In addition to these interventions, it is critical to recognise and treat the particular emotional and psychological difficulties that people with Alzheimer's disease and their carers encounter. Coping mechanisms like therapy, counselling, and support groups can offer priceless direction and emotional support all along the way.

Including supplementary and alternative self-care strategies can also improve general well-being and encourage happiness despite challenges. Acupuncture, massage, music therapy, aromatherapy, and art therapy are a few examples of these treatments. People can discover moments of joy and respite and can connect with their inner power by investigating and implementing these techniques into their daily lives.

In conclusion, one of the most important aspects of managing Alzheimer's disease is to find joy in the small things in life. People can improve their general sense of well-being and face obstacles with more resilience by implementing mindfulness exercises, gratitude exercises, and techniques for savouring happy experiences. Alzheimer's disease may be a difficult road, but with these techniques, happy, thankful, and connecting moments can be found even in the middle of the challenges.

Maintaining Independence and Autonomy

Being a physician and a health and wellness coach, I have personally witnessed the devastation that Alzheimer's disease can cause to sufferers and their families. A person's sense of identity and capacity to carry out daily chores may be progressively undermined by a progressive deterioration in cognitive function and memory loss. Nonetheless, there are strategies to enable people suffering from Alzheimer's disease to maintain their freedom and self-governance for as long as feasible.

Adaptive technologies are essential in providing people with Alzheimer's Disease with the resources they need to continue being independent. These technologies range from straightforward smartphone reminder apps to cutting-edge wearables that offer real-time vital sign monitoring and drug adherence notifications. People can use these technologies to set reminders and prompts for things like taking their medications, going to appointments, or doing self-care. In addition to promoting their freedom, these reminders lessen the load on caregivers, who could otherwise be on guard round-the-clock to make sure their loved ones are safe.

Assistive devices, in addition to adaptive technologies, play a critical role in helping people with Alzheimer's Disease live more independently. Devices that help people maintain their physical functionality and reduce the danger of accidents or injuries include grab bars in bathrooms, walking aids, and simple-to-use culinary utensils. In addition, gadgets like GPS trackers and emergency alert systems can give caregivers and the individuals they care for peace of mind by guaranteeing that assistance is close at hand in the event of an emergency or if the person wanders off.

But remaining independent and self-sufficient extends beyond using gadgets and technology. It also necessitates functional skills and a comprehensive commitment to self-care. This includes mental and emotional health as well as physical activity, diet, and overall well-being. Adopting lifestyle changes, such consistent exercise regimens catered to the person's ability, can improve physical strength and flexibility, encouraging self-sufficiency in everyday tasks like getting dressed, taking a shower, or cooking.

Preserving general health and cognitive function is also greatly aided by proper eating. Lean protein, whole grains, fruits, and vegetables are all important components of a balanced diet that can promote brain health and delay the onset of cognitive decline. Furthermore, it's critical to treat any dietary deficiencies—such as those in antioxidants, omega-3 fatty acids, and vitamins B12 and D—that may aggravate Alzheimer's disease symptoms.

Another important component of helping people with Alzheimer's disease become more independent and autonomous is counselling and psychology-related treatments. Through addressing the psychological and emotional effects of the illness, people can remain optimistic and more capable of handling life's problems. Mindfulness practises and cognitive-behavioral therapy (CBT) have demonstrated encouraging outcomes in lowering stress, anxiety, and depression while enhancing general wellbeing. These therapeutic modalities can support people with Alzheimer's disease in managing their emotions, creating useful coping mechanisms, and preserving their sense of self and identity as the condition progresses.

Moreover, coping mechanisms and self-help approaches can enable people with Alzheimer's disease to take an active role in their own care and decision-making. Encouraging people to partake in hobbies, crafts, or music can be very beneficial from a therapeutic standpoint. In addition to stimulating the mind, these activities help people feel good about themselves and like they've accomplished something. The individual can continue to partake in important and satisfying experiences by customising these activities to suit their skills and preferences.

Providing family members and caregivers with education on good communication and engagement techniques is another important aspect of empowering people with Alzheimer's disease. Simple actions that promote comprehension and reduce frustration for both parties include keeping eye contact, speaking in a soothing and quiet tone, and giving clear instructions. It is important to keep in mind that people with Alzheimer's disease could still be emotionally intelligent and have a natural desire to interact with those they love. A person's sense of autonomy and self-worth can be further enhanced by family members and caregivers by providing a compassionate and supportive atmosphere.

In summary, preserving independence and self-governance for those diagnosed with Alzheimer's Disease necessitates a multifaceted strategy that includes assistive technology, lifestyle adjustments, counselling and psychology-related approaches, self-help tactics, and efficient communication. By utilising a blend of these tactics, people can carry on with their favourite hobbies, protect their physical and mental abilities, and keep their sense of identity even as the illness advances. It is imperative to customise these tactics based on the unique requirements and capabilities of every person, guaranteeing a dignified, empowered, and purposeful journey with Alzheimer's Disease.

Building a Supportive Network

Recognizing the Need for Support

I have direct experience with the devastation that Alzheimer's disease can cause to patients and their families as a medical practitioner and health and wellness coach. A person's capacity to carry out daily chores and sense of self can be progressively undermined by a progressive deterioration in cognitive function and memory loss. To maintain their freedom and autonomy for as long as possible, people with Alzheimer's disease can, nevertheless, be empowered in certain ways.

When it comes to providing people with Alzheimer's Disease with the resources they need to continue being independent, adaptive technologies are invaluable. Simple reminder apps for cellphones or wearable technology that offers real-time vital sign monitoring and drug adherence notifications are examples of these technologies. These technologies allow people to set reminders and prompts for things like taking medication, going to appointments, or practising self-care. These prompts help them maintain their independence while also relieving caretakers of some of the load that comes with having to watch out for their loved ones all the time.

Apart from adaptive technologies, assistive devices play a crucial role in helping people with Alzheimer's Disease to live more independently. For example, equipment like culinary utensils that are simple to use, walking aids, and grab bars for toilets can assist people keep their physical functionality while lowering their risk of accidents or injuries. Additionally, by guaranteeing that assistance is close at hand in the event of an emergency or if they wander off, gadgets like GPS trackers and emergency alert systems can give folks and their caretakers peace of mind.

But remaining independent and autonomous involves more than just using gadgets and technology. Functional skills and a comprehensive commitment to self-care are also necessary. This includes everything from mental and emotional clarity to physical activity, diet, and overall health. Encouraging physical strength and flexibility through lifestyle alterations, such as customised exercise regimens, can help individuals become more independent in daily tasks like cooking, bathing, and dressing.

In addition, maintaining overall health and cognitive function is greatly aided by proper nutrition. Brain health can be supported and the rate of cognitive decline can be slowed down with a balanced diet high in fruits, vegetables, healthy grains, and lean meats. Furthermore, it is critical to treat any dietary deficiencies, such as those in omega-3 fatty acids, vitamins B12 and D, and antioxidants, that may increase Alzheimer's disease symptoms.

Another important component of encouraging independence and autonomy in people with Alzheimer's disease is counselling and psychology-related practises. People can better manage their struggles and keep a positive outlook by attending to the emotional and psychological effects of the disease. The reduction of anxiety, sadness, and stress as well as the enhancement of general well-being have been demonstrated by cognitive-behavioral therapy (CBT) and mindfulness practises. Through the course of the disease, these treatment modalities can support people with Alzheimer's disease in managing their emotions, creating useful coping mechanisms, and preserving their sense of identity.

Additionally, people with Alzheimer's Disease can be empowered to actively engage in their care and decision-making through the use of self-help approaches and coping strategies. Engaging people in hobbies, crafts, or music are examples of enjoyable activities that can have a positive therapeutic impact. Engaging in these activities not only stimulates the brain, but they also help people feel good about themselves and their achievements. These activities can be modified to accommodate the person's skills and preferences so they can carry on having satisfying experiences.

Teaching family members and caregivers efficient interaction and communication techniques is another important part of empowering people with Alzheimer's disease. Maintaining eye contact, speaking in a soothing and quiet tone, and giving precise instructions can all be small gestures that help minimise frustration and promote understanding. Remembering that people with Alzheimer's disease may still be emotionally intelligent and have a natural desire to interact with those they love is important. Caregivers and family members can further strengthen the person's sense of autonomy and self-worth by fostering a compassionate and encouraging environment.

Conclusively, preserving independence and autonomy for people diagnosed with Alzheimer's Disease necessitates an all-encompassing strategy that includes assistive technologies, adaptive technologies, lifestyle adjustments, counselling and psychology-related approaches, self-help tactics, and successful communication. By combining these tactics, people can keep doing the things they enjoy, keep their bodies and minds functioning, and keep their sense of identity intact even as their illness advances. To ensure that each person's journey with Alzheimer's Disease is filled with dignity, empowerment, and a sense of purpose, keep in mind that it is crucial to customise these tactics to each person's needs and skills.

Joining Support Groups

By joining Alzheimer's Disease support groups, you can create a network of people who are there for you when you need it most. These support groups offer a secure and compassionate space where people living with Alzheimer's disease and those supporting them can talk about their experiences, ask questions, and get advice. It can be incredibly consoling and reassuring to be surrounded by others who are experiencing comparable difficulties. In addition to offering emotional support, support groups are excellent resources for knowledge and coping mechanisms.

Seeking Community Resources

For those with Alzheimer's disease and those who care for them, communities frequently provide a variety of options. To locate the support that best meets your needs, you must look through these resources. A few community resources could be adult day care facilities, memory care facilities, transportation support, and respite care services. These services might help relieve some of the stress associated with providing care and offer caregivers a break. Furthermore, they provide an avenue for people with Alzheimer's Disease to interact with others and partake in stimulating activities, so enhancing their general well-being and quality of life.

Engaging Professional Services

To help manage Alzheimer's disease, professional services can be extremely helpful in addition to support groups and local resources. Like me, other health and wellness coaches can collaborate with patients and their carers to create individualised treatment programmes that emphasise wellness and holistic medicine. These programmes could contain recommendations for dietary and lifestyle changes, procedures connected to psychology and counselling, self-care substitutes and complementary therapies, self-help methods, and coping mechanisms. Throughout the course of Alzheimer's disease, professional services can offer continuing direction and support, enhancing the general wellbeing of both the affected person and their caregivers.

The Role of Family and Friends

Relying on friends and family for both practical and emotional support is another important part of creating a supportive network. It's critical to be transparent with loved ones on the difficulties in managing Alzheimer's disease. They may help, lend a sympathetic ear, and improve the general wellbeing of the person with Alzheimer's

Disease and their caregiver by being involved in the journey. A loving, understanding, and accepting atmosphere where the person feels loved, understood, and accepted can also be fostered by family and friends.

Self-Care and Well-being

While enlisting outside assistance is a necessary step in creating a supportive network, self-care and general wellbeing should also be prioritised. In my capacity as a physician and health and wellness advisor, I stress the need of self-care in the management of Alzheimer's disease. This entails giving adequate sleep a high priority, working out frequently, eating a balanced diet, practising mindfulness and relaxation, and cultivating healthy relationships. Taking care of oneself lowers the risk of caregiver burnout and helps caregivers deliver better care for their loved ones.

Fostering a Sense of Belonging

Creating a network of support is important for managing Alzheimer's disease, but it does more than just offer help; it helps people feel like they belong. Feelings of loneliness and isolation can be lessened by establishing connections with others who are sympathetic and aware of the difficulties presented by Alzheimer's disease. Professional services, community resources, and support groups all help to foster an atmosphere that values, comprehends, and supports people with Alzheimer's disease. Creating a sense of community is essential for preserving mental and emotional health as well as advancing a better standard of living.

Conclusion:

A key component of managing Alzheimer's disease is creating a network of support. Individuals with Alzheimer's Disease and their caregivers can better manage the challenges of the disease by acknowledging their need for support, joining support groups, looking for community resources, enlisting professional services, involving family and friends, putting self-care first, and creating a sense of community. As a physician and health and wellness coach, I place a strong emphasis on the role that a strong support system plays in advancing holistic treatment and wellness in the management of Alzheimer's disease. By working together, we can develop a comprehensive treatment plan for Alzheimer's disease that will take into account the needs of both patients and the people who care for them.

Advocacy and Empowerment

I want to provide readers the tools they need to advocate for themselves and their loved ones who have Alzheimer's in this subchapter. I'll talk about a few strategies to push for research, create awareness, and bring about positive change in dementia care. I want to use this opportunity to encourage and direct others to improve the lives of those who are impacted by this progressive neurological illness.

Increasing public knowledge about Alzheimer's disease is one of the first stages in becoming a successful advocate. The effects that this illness has on people and their families are still largely unknown to the general public. By increasing awareness of the illness and its effects, we may work to reduce the stigma attached to Alzheimer's and inform the public about the difficulties faced by persons who have the condition.

Organizing neighbourhood activities, taking part in fundraising initiatives, and making use of social media platforms are just a few ways to spread awareness. Sharing personal narratives, educational materials, and research updates are all made possible by these platforms. We can engage a larger audience and promote empathy and support for individuals with Alzheimer's by skillfully leveraging various platforms.

Supporting dementia care research is an essential component of campaigning. The remarkable progress in medical science that has illuminated the fundamental reasons and possible remedies for Alzheimer's disease has been amazing to observe. But there's still a lot of work to be done.

As advocates, we may help and promote research by funding research, taking part in clinical trials, and lending our support to organisations that conduct dementia research. We can speed up the discovery of cutting-edge treatment modalities and eventually work toward a cure by fostering a culture that appreciates and invests in research.

In addition, we need to actively engage in the policy-making process to promote positive change in dementia care. It is imperative to advocate for policies that increase funding for research, expand access to high-quality healthcare, and strengthen support services for those living with Alzheimer's disease. By interacting with legislators, we can have an impact on the creation of rules and laws that give the needs and welfare of people living with the illness first priority.

It's critical to understand that advocacy encompasses both internal and external initiatives, and that it also entails enabling Alzheimer's patients to advocate for themselves. Decision-making and communication are two areas where people with Alzheimer's disease frequently struggle. It is our duty as caregivers and healthcare providers to make sure they feel heard and given the authority to take an active role in their own care.

Person-centered care is one approach to accomplish this, as it centres decision-making around the needs and preferences of the individual and customises care plans accordingly. By integrating people with Alzheimer's in decisions about their daily routines, treatment alternatives, and care objectives, this method fosters meaningful and respectful discourse. We can improve their general well-being and give them more autonomy by encouraging a sense of empowerment.

In order to empower people with Alzheimer's and their caregivers to face the obstacles of the illness, it is also crucial to provide them with information and tools. This can include access to information on accessible support services, workshops, and support groups. We give them the information and resources they need to make wise decisions and fight for the greatest assistance and care available.

The creation of a society that supports and elevates people with Alzheimer's disease ultimately depends on advocacy and empowerment. In order to reduce the burden of dementia and enable individuals who are afflicted to live with dignity and a high quality of life, we must increase awareness, support research, and effect positive change in dementia care.

We can bring about significant change in the dementia care industry if we band together as advocates and support individuals who are impacted by Alzheimer's. Together, let's work to increase public awareness, fund research, and offer compassionate care to all those affected by Alzheimer's. We can change things and give those impacted by this terrible illness hope if we work together.

Embracing the Journey and Finding Hope

Even while hope can be difficult to come by after learning that you have Alzheimer's disease, it is a strong force that you should never undervalue. It is the glimmer of hope in the midst of hardship, the light at the end of a dark tunnel. Embracing hope allows us to be open to the possibility of a better future, even in the face of uncertainty.

But when everything around us appears to be falling apart, how can we find hope? Resilience is the key to the solution; it is the capacity to overcome adversity and adjust to changing conditions. We can stretch and contract like a rubber band, finding the fortitude to endure adversity. The ability to be resilient is a skill that can be developed by a variety of methods and approaches.

Self-compassion practise is one such method. When suffering from Alzheimer's disease, it is simple to slip into a cycle of self-criticism and blame. On the other hand, practising self-compassion entails being kind, understanding, and supportive of oneself when facing difficulties. It's about showing ourselves the same kindness we would extend to a loved one going through a comparable situation. By doing this, we cultivate an atmosphere of acceptance and forgiving inside ourselves, which enables us to face life's obstacles with more grace and resiliency.

In addition to fostering self-compassion, a holistic approach to healthcare strengthens our resilience and sense of optimism. This method entails acknowledging the connections between our mental, emotional, and physical health. It recognises that our diet, attitude, and way of living can have a significant impact on how we experience Alzheimer's disease.

In my capacity as a physician and wellness and health coach, I collaborate with a group of professionals from several wellness and health domains to offer complete care to those with Alzheimer's disease. Our emphasis is on making lifestyle changes that can enhance cognitive wellness. Regular exercise, eating a diet that supports brain health, practising mindfulness and relaxation, and participating in cognitive exercises are a few examples of these changes.

In particular, exercise is essential for fostering resilience and mental health. Studies have demonstrated that physical activity not only lowers the risk of cognitive decline and improves cardiovascular health, but it also improves cognitive performance. It promotes the synthesis of neurotrophic factors, which aid in the development and upkeep of sound brain tissue. Our ability to hope and be resilient can be enhanced, as well as our general state of well-being, by engaging in frequent exercise.

Another important factor in preserving brain health is diet. Several dietary approaches, like the Mediterranean diet, have been connected in numerous studies to a lower risk of cognitive decline and Alzheimer's disease. These diets minimise intake of processed foods, sugar, and saturated fats while emphasising the consumption of fruits, vegetables, whole grains, lean proteins, and healthy fats. We give our brains the fundamental building blocks they require for optimum functioning by feeding our bodies with nutrient-rich foods.

Furthermore, practising mindfulness and relaxation techniques to manage stress has a positive effect on our mental and emotional health. Prolonged stress not only makes Alzheimer's disease symptoms worse, but it also slows down cognitive ageing. Deep breathing exercises and other mindfulness techniques can assist to relax the mind and lower stress levels. By promoting present-moment awareness, these practises help us to find comfort in the present and release our anxieties about the past or the future.

Another crucial element of a comprehensive strategy for managing Alzheimer's disease is cognitive exercises. By strengthening memory, focus, and problem-solving abilities, these activities support the preservation and enhancement of cognitive function. They can come in many different forms, such word games, puzzles, reading, and picking up new abilities. Through these mentally demanding activities, we strengthen neural connections and encourage neuroplasticity—the brain's capacity to adapt and restructure itself, even in the face of cognitive deterioration.

It is difficult to find resilience and hope when dealing with Alzheimer's disease. It calls for fortitude, tenacity, and an openness to unpredictability. However, we may handle this difficult path with dignity and grace if we practise self-compassion, embrace a holistic approach to treatment, and make lifestyle changes. Never forget that you are not travelling alone. Seek the advice of healthcare specialists who can offer you the required tools and techniques to help you find resilience and hope, as well as support from others and your loved ones.

Chapter 6: Resources and Support for Alzheimer's Disease

National and International Alzheimer's Organizations

1. Alzheimer's Association (United States)

Leading American nonprofit, the Alzheimer's Association works to improve brain health, support afflicted people and their families, and further research. They offer an abundance of services, such as a trained professional-staffed 24/7 Helpline that provides discreet help and information. In a number of locations, the organisation offers community events, educational workshops, and support groups. They also support policy modifications and offer financial support for innovative research.

2. Alzheimer's Society (United Kingdom)

The largest research and support organisation in the UK for people with dementia is the Alzheimer's Society. Through their online community and helpline, they offer guidance and support, as well as resources and information to assist individuals understand dementia and its effects. The organisation also provides funding for studies and educational initiatives aimed at raising public knowledge about Alzheimer's disease.

3. Alzheimer's Disease International (ADI)

Alzheimer's Disease International is an international federation of national and international Alzheimer's groups. In addition to assisting and working with national Alzheimer's societies, ADI advances the rights and general welfare of individuals suffering from dementia. Their main goals are to improve care and support systems around the world by expanding research, increasing public awareness, and promoting the creation of policies.

4. The Global Alzheimer's & Dementia Action Alliance (GADAA)

GADAA is an international alliance dedicated to promoting action and transformation to enhance the quality of life for those with dementia and to address the issues that face their carers worldwide. Leading Alzheimer's organisations, activists, and specialists come together through the alliance to collaborate on a common goal. They seek to improve funding and innovation in research and care, elevate the voices of those impacted by Alzheimer's disease, and have an impact on practise and policy.

5. Alzheimer Society of Canada

Support is available for both carers and patients with Alzheimer's disease and related dementias from the Alzheimer Society of Canada. Across the nation, they provide workshops, counselling, support groups, and educational resources. In an effort to enhance the lives of persons affected by the illness, the group also supports policy changes and provides funding for research.

6. Alzheimer's Australia

The leading organisation in Australia advocating for the rights of people with dementia is Alzheimer's Australia. To assist people in navigating the dementia journey, the organisation provides information resources, instructional programmes, and support services. Additionally, they support research to better understand and treat Alzheimer's disease and push for a culture that is dementia-friendly.

7. The Alzheimer's Foundation of America (AFA)

A nonprofit organisation called the Alzheimer's Foundation of America offers assistance, programmes, and information to people with Alzheimer's disease as well as to their family and carers. They run a toll-free hotline staffed by certified social workers and provide workshops and instructional programmes all across the country. Additionally, the organisation supports federal funding increases for Alzheimer's disease research.

8. Alzheimer's Society of India

An non-governmental organisation called the Alzheimer's Society of India works to raise awareness and provide assistance for people in India who are affected by dementias, including Alzheimer's disease. In order to assist those impacted by the illness, they provide counselling services, caregiver support groups, and educational programmes. Their goal is to provide comprehensive care and support services to enhance the quality of life for individuals with dementia and those who are caring for them.

9. Alzheimer Europe

A nonprofit group called Alzheimer Europe works to enhance the quality of life for Europeans who are caring for a loved one who has dementia. They support and assist people with Alzheimer's disease and their families by offering information, resources, and assistance in a variety of languages. In order to develop research agendas and policies that meet the needs of people affected by dementia, the organisation also collaborates closely with legislators and scientists.

10. The Lewy Body Dementia Association (LBDA)

A nonprofit organisation called the Lewy Body Dementia Association assists people with Lewy body dementia (LBD), their families, and medical professionals. Their main objectives are to increase public knowledge of LBD, encourage research endeavours, and offer instructional materials that facilitate prompt and precise diagnosis. The society also provides educational conferences and support groups to assist people with dementia and their caregivers in overcoming the particular difficulties brought on by this particular kind of dementia.

In conclusion, people with Alzheimer's disease and their carers have access to a vital network of resources and support because to the existence of both national and worldwide Alzheimer's organisations. These groups are essential in educating the public, sponsoring research, campaigning for policy changes, and increasing awareness. We may make great progress toward comprehensive Alzheimer's disease management and, eventually, a world free from the grip of this debilitating disorder by utilising their combined knowledge and experience.

Online Communities and Support Groups

The internet has become an essential component of our everyday life in the current digital era. It has completely changed how we interact, communicate, and look for information. Alzheimer's disease-focused online forums and support groups have grown to be invaluable tools for those afflicted with the crippling illness and their families. These online communities provide a sense of belonging, comprehension, and assistance that can be immensely beneficial in overcoming the obstacles associated with having Alzheimer's disease.

The ability to interact with people going through similar situations is one of the main advantages of online forums and support groups. When someone with Alzheimer's disease is diagnosed, they and their loved ones frequently experience feelings of loneliness and isolation. By joining an online community, they can find comfort in the knowledge that they are not travelling alone and can share their experiences, worries, and fears in a safe and supportive environment.

These online communities also provide a plethora of resources and information. Access to research papers, articles, and professional guidance on subjects ranging from the newest medical procedures and drugs to useful advise for handling daily chores is available to members. People can feel empowered by this information and be better able to make decisions regarding their treatment. Online communities also frequently arrange webinars, live chats, and Q&A sessions with medical specialists, giving participants the chance to ask questions and learn from subject matter experts.

Engaging in virtual communities or support groups can also provide favourable effects on one's mental health and overall wellbeing. Alzheimer's disease is a degenerative illness that can lead to severe mental suffering in both the afflicted person and those who provide care for them. It may be very healing to be able to ask for help, share stories, and assist others. It can ease tension, give one a sense of purpose and belonging, and lessen feelings of loneliness.

Online forums and support groups can provide helpful guidance and coping mechanisms in addition to emotional support. Members can exchange experiences and get knowledge from others about how to successfully communicate, manage symptoms, and preserve a good standard of living. The combined knowledge of these communities is extensive and varied, ranging from routines and memory help creation advice to methods for keeping an active lifestyle.

Selecting trustworthy platforms that put privacy and security first is crucial when looking for online forums and support groups. Because personal information shared in these groups is sensitive, make sure the platform you select has strong privacy settings and complies with data protection laws. Joining communities or organisations run by healthcare experts is also a good idea since they can act as a kind of watchdog and make sure that discussions are civil, educational, and encouraging.

The online community of the Alzheimer's Association is a well-known resource for support on Alzheimer's disease. It is a dependable option for anyone looking for direction and connection because of its solid reputation and dedication to offering accurate information and help. The Alzheimer's Society's Talking Point forum is another reliable resource. It provides a secure environment where those impacted by Alzheimer's Disease can talk about their experiences and get support from others who are aware of the difficulties they encounter.

In conclusion, people with Alzheimer's disease and their families can find a great deal of information, connection, and support via online forums and support groups. These online communities foster empathy and camaraderie, lessen feelings of loneliness, and provide people the tools they need to take charge of their own care. People can obtain professional guidance and acquire coping mechanisms from others who have experienced similar circumstances thanks to the abundance of resources at their disposal. It is crucial to select trustworthy platforms that give privacy and security first priority when looking for these communities. We can establish a network of empowerment and support for individuals impacted by Alzheimer's Disease by utilising technology.

Caregiver Resources and Respite Care Options

I have worked directly with individuals and families afflicted by Alzheimer's Disease in my capacity as a physician and health and wellness coach. The assistance and break required for caregivers is one facet of their care that is frequently disregarded. Providing care for a loved one afflicted with Alzheimer's disease is an emotionally and physically taxing job. Access to resources that can offer caregivers the assistance and relief they require is crucial.

In this section, I'll go over some helpful resources for caregivers and options for respite care that can help people and families deal with the challenges of Alzheimer's disease. The aforementioned services and solutions are designed to offer caregivers the assistance, knowledge, and short-term respite they require to preserve their own physical and mental health.

1. Alzheimer's Association: A vital resource for those who look after someone who has Alzheimer's disease is the Alzheimer's Association. They provide a range of services, such as a helpline that is open around-the-clock, instructional resources, and support groups. Caregivers can connect, share stories, and get assistance from others going through similar struggles in support groups. Caretakers can better traverse the different stages of Alzheimer's disease and comprehend the disease's course with the aid of educational materials. For caretakers, the round-the-clock helpline is a lifeline, providing direction and assistance when required.

2. Local support groups: Numerous local towns have their own support groups designed especially for caregivers of people with Alzheimer's Disease in addition to the Alzheimer's Association. These support groups, which frequently get together on a regular basis, allow caregivers a secure place to talk about their experiences, get guidance,

and get emotional support. For caregivers looking to establish connections and create a support system within their community, local support groups are a great tool.

3. Respite care services: The purpose of respite care services is to offer professional care for family members suffering from Alzheimer's disease, thereby temporarily relieving caregivers. The duration of this care might vary from a few hours to many days, giving caregivers the chance to relax, take care of personal matters, or just refuel. There are several places where respite care can be offered, such as residential institutions, adult day care centres, or in-home care. It is imperative that caregivers look into the respite care choices in their community because this service can significantly reduce the strain of providing care and help caregivers avoid burnout.

4. Adult day care centers: Adult day care centres offer interesting activities and supervised care for people with cognitive impairments, including Alzheimer's disease. These facilities provide a stimulating and comfortable atmosphere where people with Alzheimer's disease can interact with others and take part in activities catered to their ability. In addition to offering caregivers a break from their caregiving responsibilities, adult day care facilities make sure that their loved ones are getting the proper attention and stimulation in a monitored environment. During this period of time off, caregivers can take care of their own needs, perform errands, or just relax.

5. In-home care services: Caregivers who want assistance and care in the comfort of their own homes can employ specialists through in-home care services. These specialists have received training in helping people with Alzheimer's disease with activities of daily living, including clothing, taking care of their medications, bathing, and cooking. Depending on the needs of the individual, in-home care services might take the form of a few hours a day or round the clock assistance. Employing in-home care gives caregivers a momentary

reprieve while guaranteeing that their loved ones receive individualised attention in a setting they are accustomed to.

6. Family and friends: The influence of their personal support system should not be undervalued by caregivers. A family's and friends' support and brief relief can be a priceless resource. Families with Alzheimer's disease can rely on their loved ones to help with caregiving responsibilities or just to spend time with them, providing the caregiver with a much-needed break. It is imperative that carers let their support system know what they need and that they are willing to receive assistance. Caregivers can prevent burnout and preserve their personal wellbeing by delegating some of the caregiving duties to others.

In conclusion, assistance, information, and short-term respite are necessary for caregivers of people with Alzheimer's disease to overcome their obstacles. The Alzheimer's Association, neighbourhood support groups, adult day care facilities, in-home care services, respite care services, and the assistance of family and friends are just a few of the resources and options for caregiving that have been covered in this section. In order to maintain their own well-being while providing care for their loved ones with Alzheimer's Disease, caregivers can receive the support and relief they need by making use of these services and opportunities. Keep in mind that carers also require care.

Financial and Legal Planning

It can be difficult to deal with a loved one's Alzheimer's diagnosis on an emotional and practical level. People may suffer from memory loss, cognitive impairment, and trouble with everyday tasks as the illness worsens. Their capacity to handle their money and make judgments may be significantly impacted by this. Proactive financial and legal planning is therefore necessary to guarantee that the individual suffering from Alzheimer's disease and their loved ones are suitably equipped for the future.

Gaining a thorough grasp of one's present financial circumstances is the first stage in financial planning. Obtaining data on their earnings, outlays, possessions, and debts is part of this. In order to evaluate the available financial resources and create a realistic budget, speaking with an accountant or financial counsellor may be beneficial. This can lessen financial strain and guarantee that there are enough resources to pay for support and care services.

It is imperative to take care of the legal issues related to Alzheimer's disease in addition to financial planning. This entails creating the required legal documentation to guarantee that the individual's desires are honoured and their rights are safeguarded. A living will, a healthcare proxy, and a durable power of attorney are the three most crucial legal instruments.

A durable power of attorney gives the person with Alzheimer's disease the authority to appoint someone to handle their financial affairs. This guarantees that even in the event that they are unable to manage their financial affairs alone, they can. It is essential to choose a reliable individual who can act in the person's best interest and make wise financial judgments.

The terms "living will" and "advance directive" refer to a document that expresses a person's desires regarding their medical care and final arrangements. Their desires for life-sustaining therapies and medical procedures are honoured thanks to this agreement. To make sure that the document appropriately captures the person's current preferences and values, it is crucial to have these discussions early on and to revisit them on a regular basis.

A person who can make medical choices on behalf of an individual with Alzheimer's disease is designated by a healthcare proxy, which is also referred to as a healthcare power of attorney. This person is in charge of speaking out for their healthcare requirements and making sure they get the right kind of attention and care. The individual chosen must be able to interact with healthcare professionals and comprehend the patient's values and preferences.

It is crucial to take into account additional legal factors in addition to these legal documents, such as estate planning, qualifying for government assistance, and long-term care insurance. Financial peace of mind can be obtained by purchasing long-term care insurance, which can assist in defraying the expense of care in a nursing home or assisted living facility.

Alzheimer's patients may also be eligible for government benefits like Medicaid and Social Security Disability Insurance. Both access to healthcare services and financial support are possible through these initiatives. To ascertain eligibility and handle the application process, speak with a Medicaid planning specialist financial advisor or elder law attorney.

Another essential part of legal and financial preparation for Alzheimer's disease is estate planning. This entails naming beneficiaries for assets such bank accounts, investments, and real estate as well as drafting a will and establishing a trust. Estate planning can assist avoid tax effects and guarantees that an individual's assets are dispersed in accordance with their desires.

Investigating the resources and support services accessible to people with Alzheimer's disease and their families is crucial, in addition to the previously stated actions. These resources can offer helpful advice, support, and information all along the path of treating the illness. Online forums, support groups, and local Alzheimer's societies can all be great places to find information and assistance.

Although legal and financial preparation may seem intimidating, these components may be successfully navigated with the correct help and advice. Early preparation and involvement of all pertinent parties—such as the Alzheimer's patient, their family, healthcare providers, financial advisors, and legal experts—are essential. Together, we can develop a thorough plan that safeguards the person's financial stability, upholds their legal rights, and gives their family peace of mind.

This subchapter concludes by discussing the critical role that legal and financial preparation plays in the management of Alzheimer's disease. We've talked about the importance of early planning, the necessary legal paperwork, and the different financial and legal factors related to the illness. Individuals and their families affected by Alzheimer's disease can effectively manage these obstacles and maintain order in their financial and legal matters by following the appropriate procedures and utilising the tools that are accessible. Keep in mind that there are experts and support services available to help you at every stage of this journey; you are not alone.

Assistive Technologies and Adaptive Devices

I have always stressed the value of holistic healthcare and wellbeing as a medical practitioner and health and wellness coach. I work with a lot of people who have Alzheimer's disease, so I am aware of how important it is to improve their independence and quality of life. This subsection delves into assistive technology and adaptive gadgets that have the potential to significantly improve the quality of life for individuals afflicted with Alzheimer's disease. I'll go over a number of resources and offer suggestions for getting access to these useful resources.

The purpose of assistive technologies is to help people do tasks that have become difficult because of cognitive deterioration. These technologies, which can be as basic as gadgets or as sophisticated as entire systems, are all meant to facilitate independence and ease daily tasks. A reminder system is one such tool that can be quite helpful for those with Alzheimer's who have memory loss. These systems may take the shape of a wearable gadget, voice-activated assistant, or smartphone app. These tools help people maintain a feeling of routine and lessen worry by offering timely reminders for crucial tasks, appointments, and medication.

A GPS tracking gadget is another useful piece of assistive technology for those with Alzheimer's. Those suffering with this illness frequently wander, which can be very dangerous. Incorporating GPS tracking devices into commonplace items like watches, shoes, or clothing enables loved ones and caretakers to find the person in the event that they become lost. This technology guarantees the person's safety in addition to giving caregivers piece of mind.

Conversely, adaptive gadgets are specially made instruments that let people do things more quickly and on their own. These gadgets support a number of daily life activities, including personal care, communication, and mobility. A walking assistance is one of these gadgets; examples include powered wheelchairs, rollators, and walking sticks. With the steadiness and assistance these tools offer, people can confidently move through their environment. The right walking assistance might be suggested to increase mobility and lower the risk of falls, depending on the person's physical capabilities and the stage of Alzheimer's.

Since language and articulation are frequently affected by the advancement of Alzheimer's disease, communication devices are especially crucial for those who have the disease. For those in the later stages of the disease, augmentative and alternative communication (AAC) technologies can be very helpful in aiding conversation. These tools might be as basic as picture boards or communication books, or they can be as complex as sophisticated computer gadgets that can speak text to speech. AAC devices give people a way to express themselves, which helps them interact with others and their environment.

People with Alzheimer's disease may find it difficult to provide for themselves, but adaptive technology can make life much easier. For instance, long-handled brushes or combs are examples of assistive technology that can make it simpler for people to take care of themselves on their own. Similarly, persons with motor impairments can feed themselves more easily with the use of adaptive eating utensils. These modest but useful gadgets help people with Alzheimer's feel more autonomous and dignified.

Now that we know how important adaptive devices and assistive technologies are, let's look at some resources and suggestions for using them. The Alzheimer's Association is one such site that offers a plethora of knowledge and assistance to both patients and caregivers. They provide assistance in locating nearby resources, such as businesses that specialise in the distribution of assistive technology. The Alzheimer's Association can also put people in touch with their local chapter so they can take advantage of support groups and educational opportunities to improve their knowledge and use of assistive technologies.

Healthcare providers and experts that specialise in Alzheimer's care are another important resource. These experts can offer advice on how to use and maintain adapted devices and assistive technology in addition to making recommendations. They might be in partnerships or contact with the vendors or producers of these products, which might make the acquisition process easier.

Another great way to get assistive technologies and adaptable equipment is an online marketplace or specialised business that serves people with impairments. There are many different items available on websites like AbleData and Independent Living Centers, along with thorough product details and user reviews. As a result, people and caregivers can decide what's best for them depending on their individual requirements and preferences.

Finally, it's critical to confirm with insurance companies because some adaptive devices and assistive technology may be paid for by health insurance policies. Furthermore, government or nonprofit groups may offer grants or funding schemes that might help defray the cost of these gadgets.

In summary, adaptive technology and assistive technologies have the power to change the lives of people with Alzheimer's by preserving their freedom and standard of living. People can maintain their sense of control over their lives and their enjoyment of the things they enjoy by implementing these tools into their everyday routines. Never forget that in order to make sure the best assistive technologies and adaptive devices are chosen for each individual's particular needs, it is imperative to ask for help and look into a variety of resources.

Research Studies and Clinical Trials

I sincerely believe in the power of research and the significance of keeping up with the most recent developments in the management of Alzheimer's disease as a medical practitioner and health and wellness coach. I have seen directly through my work the positive impact that clinical trials and research studies may have on patients' and their families' lives. Not only do these research further scientific understanding, but they also give hope to those who are impacted by Alzheimer's.

Numerous advantages can result from taking part in clinical trials and research investigations. Above all, it makes state-of-the-art therapies and interventions accessible to people that might not be possible through traditional medical care. Individuals who participate in trials may benefit from the ongoing research into new medications, treatments, and treatment approaches aimed at improving our understanding of and ability to treat Alzheimer's disease.

Individuals can also actively contribute to scientific knowledge and breakthroughs by taking part in research projects and clinical trials. By contributing to our growing understanding of the condition, each participant helps to open the door to better therapies and, eventually, an Alzheimer's disease cure. People constitute an essential component of the worldwide effort to fight this terrible sickness by contributing their voices and experiences to research.

Research studies and clinical trials provide a special support system for participants in addition to possible rewards. Experts from a variety of health and wellness sectors work in multidisciplinary teams to perform these studies. Specialists such as neurologists, psychologists, dietitians, and social workers who offer comprehensive care and support during the study are available for collaboration with participants. Participants will receive individualised attention and a thorough treatment plan that takes into account every facet of their well-being thanks to this holistic approach to healthcare.

Although locating pertinent research studies and clinical trials might be difficult, there are many tools available to make the process easier. An reputable institution devoted to Alzheimer's Disease research, advocacy, and support is the Alzheimer's Association. On their website, users can search a database of current trials and studies and filter results based on criteria including geography, age eligibility, and research objectives.

A comprehensive global registry of clinical studies, clinicaltrials.gov is another invaluable resource. People can look up Alzheimer's disease-related trials using this easy-to-use database, which offers comprehensive details about the goals, requirements, and contact details of each study. Through the use of these tools, people can access a multitude of knowledge and opportunities related to research participation.

It is essential to carefully weigh the advantages, dangers, and obligations of any research project or clinical trial before deciding to participate. Ensuring that participants have a comprehensive comprehension of the study's objectives, protocols, and any adverse effects is a crucial aspect of ethical research through informed consent. In order to make an informed choice that fits with one's unique needs and objectives, it is critical to communicate openly and ask questions of the research team.

Keeping in mind that involvement in clinical trials and research studies is completely voluntary is also crucial. People have the freedom to decline participation at any moment and should never feel pressured to do so. The choice to take part should be made after giving serious thought to one's preferences, circumstances, and advice from medical experts.

It's crucial to keep in mind that while taking part in clinical trials and research studies can be an effective strategy for managing

Alzheimer's disease, they are only one aspect of the jigsaw. Individuals can improve their overall well-being and empower themselves in the face of Alzheimer's Disease by incorporating coping strategies, food and diet planning, counselling and psychology-related techniques, various self-care alternative and complimentary techniques, self-help techniques, and lifestyle modifications into their daily lives.

In conclusion, there is a window of opportunity for those impacted by Alzheimer's Disease thanks to scientific studies and clinical trials. By taking part in these trials, people can obtain state-of-the-art therapies, advance scientific understanding, and receive a strong network of support. Accessible tools like clinicaltrials.gov and the Alzheimer's Association make it easier to locate pertinent possibilities. Making decisions based on individual circumstances and preferences requires thorough understanding of the advantages, hazards, and requirements associated with involvement. People can maximise their well-being and take charge of their own care by incorporating a holistic approach to managing Alzheimer's disease.

Books, Websites, and Further Reading

Books:

1. "The Alzheimer's Prevention & Treatment Diet" by Dr. Richard S. Isaacson

The well-known neurologist and expert on Alzheimer's disease, Dr. Isaacson, explores the relationship between nutrition and cognitive function in this book. In order to assist prevent and treat Alzheimer's Disease, he offers scientific proof, useful advice, and a customised approach to nutrition.

2. "The 36-Hour Day: Nancy L. Mace and Peter V. Rabins' "A Family Guide to Caring for People with Alzheimer Disease, Other Dementias, and Memory Loss in Later Life"

- For relatives and caregivers of people with Alzheimer's disease, this book is a vital resource. It includes tips for handling difficult behaviours, communication and care tactics, and helpful advice.

3. "Still Alice" by Lisa Genova

- Despite not being a nonfiction work, "Still Alice" offers a moving and perceptive portrait of life with early-onset Alzheimer's. Readers are given further insight into the psychological and personal effects of the illness from Alice, the main character's, perspective.

4. "The Gene: An Intimate History" by Siddhartha Mukherjee

While not only concentrating on Alzheimer's disease, "The Gene" offers an extensive investigation into genetics and their function in the emergence of several ailments, including Alzheimer's. This book provides insightful information about the science underlying the illness and a wider viewpoint.

Websites:

1. Alzheimer's Association (www.alz.org)

- For those with Alzheimer's disease and their families, the Alzheimer's Association is a reliable source of advocacy, information, and support. Their website provides a plethora of knowledge regarding the illness, developments in the field, available treatments, and support resources.

2. National Institute on Aging (www.nia.nih.gov/alzheimers)

One excellent resource for learning about Alzheimer's disease and related dementias is the National Institute on Aging, which is a division of the National Institutes of Health. Comprehensive resources, such as research articles, instructional materials, and details on clinical trials, are available on their website.

3. Alzheimer's Research UK (www.alzheimersresearchuk.org)

- Alzheimer's Research UK provides a plethora of information about research developments, fundraising campaigns, and support programmes for readers looking for a global viewpoint. To remain informed about the most recent developments and efforts in Alzheimer's research, visit their website, which is a great resource.

4. Mayo Clinic (www.mayoclinic.org/diseases-conditions/ alzheimers-disease)

- The Mayo Clinic is well known for its knowledge and all-encompassing approach to medicine. Their website provides a dependable and easy-to-use resource for information on Alzheimer's disease, including diagnosis, treatment alternatives, and suggested lifestyle changes.

Additional Resources:

1. Alzheimer's Disease Research Foundation

- This organisation is committed to providing funding for studies that seek to identify the underlying causes of Alzheimer's disease, create efficient therapies, and eventually discover a cure. On their website, you may find out about their ongoing clinical trials, research initiatives, and opportunities to support their purpose by becoming involved.

2. Alzheimer's Society

- The Alzheimer's Society is an organisation situated in the United Kingdom that offers a variety of support services to people with Alzheimer's disease and their families. Their website provides tools, information, and a helpline for people in need of direction and assistance.

3. "Ask the Expert" Webinars

- A number of respectable institutions, like the Mayo Clinic and the Alzheimer's Association, provide webinars with knowledgeable presenters that cover different facets of Alzheimer's disease. These webinars offer the chance to hear from top experts and ask targeted questions about the illness.

4. Support Groups

For those with Alzheimer's disease and those who care for them, joining a support group can be extremely beneficial in terms of both practical advice and emotional support. Hospitals, community centres, and Alzheimer's Associations in the area frequently lead support groups that offer a secure setting for people to interact and exchange stories about comparable struggles.

Keep in mind that information is power as you begin your adventure with Alzheimer's disease. The recommended books, websites, and supplementary materials will prove to be invaluable tools and allies along your journey through the intricacies of the illness. Always seek advice from your healthcare physician and use these resources in addition to expert advice for a thorough and all-encompassing strategy to managing Alzheimer's disease.

Helplines and Emergency Contacts

It might be challenging to know where to turn in a crisis. For this reason, I have put together a list of emergency numbers and helplines that are specifically dedicated to Alzheimer's disease and related matters. These services are committed to provide direction, encouragement, and prompt help to people and their caregivers, and they are accessible around-the-clock:

1. Alzheimer's Association Helpline: One of the top organisations for Alzheimer's support, care, and research is the Alzheimer's Association. Their helpline provides trustworthy information, assistance, and emotional support to people with Alzheimer's disease and those who are caring for them. The skilled experts on the other end of the line can help with a variety of issues, from comprehending the course of the illness to offering solutions for difficult behaviours.

2. Alzheimer's Foundation of America Helpline: For those who have Alzheimer's and their families, the Alzheimer's Foundation of America is yet another priceless resource. Their helpline connects people to local resources by offering assistance, information, and referral services. The helpline is available to provide direction and support, regardless of the need for help locating support groups or obtaining healthcare treatments.

3. Eldercare Locator: A national resource that helps older people and their carers find local services and resources is the Eldercare Locator. From respite care services to community-based support programmes, they can help find it all. Their helpline is a great resource for people with Alzheimer's and their families, guiding them through the very challenging world of providing care.

4. National Suicide Prevention Lifeline: Providing care for an individual with Alzheimer's disease can be emotionally taxing and burdensome. It's critical to focus and take care of your mental health. Free, private help is available via the National Suicide Prevention

Lifeline to anybody in need, including those who are looking after someone who has Alzheimer's. They have skilled specialists on duty around-the-clock to staff their helpline and provide support, encouragement, and guidance to those in need.

5. Crisis Text Line: Finding the right words to convey your feelings during a crisis might be difficult at times. Through text messaging, The Crisis Text Line connects those in need of instant support with qualified crisis counsellors who are available to offer advice and a listening ear. Texting the Crisis Text Line can be a lifesaver when you're feeling overwhelmed or need someone to talk to.

6. Local Support Groups: Utilizing local support networks is crucial in addition to national resources and helplines. Local support groups for Alzheimer's patients can offer a secure setting for people to interact with one another through comparable experiences. These support groups provide information, emotional support, and helpful guidance from people who have personal experience with the difficulties of caring for an Alzheimer's patient. To locate local support groups, get in touch with the Alzheimer's Association or community centres.

7. Emergency Services: It is essential to have access to nearby emergency services in case of a medical emergency or other dire circumstances. Make sure you always have the phone numbers of the fire department, police department, and ambulance service close at hand. In an emergency, having rapid access to emergency services helps guarantee timely assistance.

Never forget that you are not travelling alone. You have access to an enormous support system. If you have any queries or need support, don't hesitate to contact these hotlines and emergency contacts. The wellbeing of both you and your loved one suffering from Alzheimer's disease is crucial, and these tools are designed to support you as you work through any obstacles that may arise.

Having a network of friends, family, and medical experts who can offer support and direction is crucial, in addition to these hotlines and emergency contacts. Never forget to put self-care first, ask for expert assistance when necessary, and rely on your loved ones for support. It is possible to manage the difficulties associated with Alzheimer's disease and give yourself and your loved one the best care possible if you have access to the appropriate tools and a robust support system.

Chapter 7: The Future of Alzheimer's Disease Management

Advances in Early Detection and Diagnosis

A potentially useful technique for the early diagnosis of Alzheimer's disease is the use of biomarkers. These are quantifiable biological markers that can offer important information about the occurrence and course of the illness. Amyloid-beta, a protein that deposits as plaques in the brains of Alzheimer's patients, is one such biomarker. Scientists can assess amyloid-beta levels and identify whether there is an excess present, suggesting the presence of the disease, through the use of blood tests or cerebrospinal fluid testing. Since high levels of tau are linked to the neurofibrillary tangles that characterise Alzheimer's disease, tau protein has also showed potential as a biomarker. Through the examination of these biomarkers, it may be possible to diagnose the illness before symptoms become apparent.

Recent advancements in neuroimaging techniques have also made it possible for us to see the anatomy and function of the brain in previously unheard-of detail. Although magnetic resonance imaging (MRI) has long been used to examine the brain, new advancements in the field have made MRI even more useful for Alzheimer's disease early detection. Changes in the structure of the brain, such as the shrinking of the hippocampus, which is important for memory and learning, can be seen using high-resolution MRI images. This shrinking is frequently a precursor to Alzheimer's. Moreover, functional magnetic resonance imaging (fMRI) can shed light on patterns of brain activity by highlighting regions of decreased activity that can be suggestive of a disease. These neuroimaging methods assist distinguish Alzheimer's from other types of dementia in addition to helping detect the disease early.

Novel diagnostic instruments have also surfaced, providing fresh perspectives on early Alzheimer's disease detection. Using virtual reality (VR) technology to evaluate cognitive function is one such tool. We can assess patients' cognitive capacities in a more engaging and realistic way by immersing them in virtual environments and assigning them different activities. This can give important details regarding any possible cognitive impairment, which can aid in the early detection of Alzheimer's. Furthermore, smartphone apps have been created to help with Alzheimer's early detection. Through a variety of tests and exams, these apps gather information on a user's cognitive capacities, enabling routine monitoring and prompt intervention in the event that a decrease is noticed. Early detection of Alzheimer's disease can now be easily and conveniently done with the help of these cutting-edge diagnostic instruments.

Even while these developments in early diagnosis and detection are very encouraging, it's crucial to keep in mind that they are only one aspect of an all-encompassing strategy for managing Alzheimer's disease. Alzheimer's patients and their loved ones may find the diagnosis to be daunting, so it's important to support and mentor them through the process. I'm dedicated to providing my patients with holistic healthcare and wellness as a medical doctor and health and wellness coach. My team comprises professionals from other health and wellness domains, with whom I collaborate to offer an all-encompassing strategy for managing Alzheimer's disease. In order to address the emotional and psychological aspects of the disease, this includes dietary and lifestyle adjustments including exercise as well as counselling and psychology techniques. To enable people to take an active role in their own treatment, we also include self-help approaches, coping mechanisms, and alternative and complementary forms of self-care.

In conclusion, there is hope for early intervention and better disease management due to the advancements in the early identification and diagnosis of Alzheimer's disease. Innovative diagnostic tools, neuroimaging methods, and biomarkers offer important insights into the onset and course of Alzheimer's disease, enabling early detection and treatment. But it's important to keep in mind that these developments are only a small portion of an all-encompassing strategy for managing Alzheimer's disease. Through the integration of these early detection techniques with a comprehensive approach to healthcare and wellbeing, we can provide Alzheimer's patients and their families with the necessary support and direction to effectively navigate this difficult journey.

Precision Medicine and Personalized Treatment Approaches

Precision medicine has found use for genetic testing as a useful tool. We can now determine which genetic changes may raise an individual's risk of Alzheimer's Disease with a straightforward genetic test. A increased risk of the disease has been linked to the existence of specific genes, such as the apolipoprotein E (APOE) gene. Through the identification of these genetic markers, individuals can receive tailored interventions aimed at lowering their risk or delaying the advancement of their disease, in addition to receiving a more accurate risk assessment.

Another essential element of precision medicine in the treatment of Alzheimer's disease is biomarker analysis. Biomarkers are quantifiable indicators of bodily biological processes. When it comes to Alzheimer's disease, some biomarkers can be used to detect aberrant proteins like tau and beta-amyloid that are linked to the illness. We are able to track the evolution of Alzheimer's disease and its response to treatment by assessing these biomarkers using different imaging techniques like positron emission tomography (PET) or cerebrospinal fluid analysis. This allows us to diagnose Alzheimer's disease earlier.

Personalized therapy approaches can be designed if a thorough understanding of an individual's genetic predisposition and biomarker profile has been obtained. When it comes to managing Alzheimer's disease, there is no one size fits all approach. By customising interventions to meet each patient's specific needs, we can increase treatment efficacy and enhance quality of life.

A tailored strategy that can be used is changing one's lifestyle. Diet, exercise, sleep habits, and stress reduction are examples of lifestyle variables that have a big impact on brain health and can affect how quickly a disease progresses. We are able to pinpoint particular areas of concern and suggest focused lifestyle improvements to maximise brain health by examining an individual's genetic and biomarker profile. For instance, if genetic testing indicates a higher risk of brain inflammation, we would suggest an anti-inflammatory diet high in antioxidants, omega-3 fatty acids, and turmeric. In a similar vein, in order to improve brain waste clearance, we would advise boosting physical activity and encouraging a regular sleep schedule if biomarker data shows a drop in amyloid clearance.

Techniques from psychology and counselling are also essential components of customised Alzheimer's disease treatment plans. Emotionally taxing living with the illness can be on the patient as well as their loved ones and caregivers. The emotional and psychological components of Alzheimer's Disease can be managed by individuals and their families with the help of counselling and psychology-related treatments like mindfulness-based stress reduction, cognitive-behavioral therapy, and support groups. These methods can lessen anxiety, elevate wellbeing overall, and boost mood.

Personalized treatment plans may involve complementary and alternative therapies in addition to psychological support and lifestyle changes. These treatments, which include aromatherapy, music therapy, acupuncture, and herbal cures, can be customised to meet the unique needs and symptoms of each patient. For instance, if someone is having trouble sleeping, we might look into using sound therapy or lavender essential oil to help them relax and have a better night's sleep. It is crucial to remember that although complementary and alternative therapies might offer extra assistance, they should always be utilised in addition to traditional medical care.

Another important element of individualised Alzheimer's disease treatment plans is the use of self-help techniques. With the aid of these strategies, people can feel more in control of their everyday life and be empowered to actively participate in their own management. Self-help methods might include stress reduction strategies like deep breathing exercises and guided visualisation, as well as memory-boosting activities and brain training applications. People can boost their general well-being, lessen stress, and improve cognitive performance by adopting these practises into their regular routines.

Finally, the individual's particular circumstances and preferences should be taken into account while developing a personalised treatment plan. Since everyone is affected by Alzheimer's disease differently, what works for one person might not work for another. We can make certain that the treatment plan is not only successful but also in line with the goals and values of the patient by actively including them in the decision-making process and taking their preferences into account. This method encourages a collaborative relationship between the patient and the healthcare professional as well as patient-centered care.

In summary, individualised treatment plans and precision medicine have completely changed the way that Alzheimer's disease is managed. We can now provide targeted therapies, biomarker analysis, and genetic testing to optimise illness management through customised treatment programmes. These approaches cater to the specific needs of each individual and enable them to actively participate in their own health, ranging from lifestyle modifications and counselling to alternative therapies and self-help strategies. We are getting closer to a day when Alzheimer's Disease can be successfully treated and lives positively touched by advances in our knowledge and use of precision medicine.

Emerging Therapies and Disease-Modifying Treatments

The search for Alzheimer's disease therapies that alter the condition has attracted a lot of scientific attention lately. The main goals of conventional disease management strategies have been to reduce symptoms and delay the rate at which cognitive impairment is occurring. On the other hand, new treatments try to address the fundamental causes of Alzheimer's in an effort to slow down or even reverse the progression of the illness. This signifies a substantial change in our strategy and gives millions of people and their families affected by this terrible neurological illness hope.

Immunotherapy is one of the most exciting areas of Alzheimer's disease research. Immunotherapies function by using the immune system of the body to target and eliminate aberrant proteins that are indicative of Alzheimer's disease, such as tau tangles and amyloid-beta plaques. It is thought that these aberrant proteins are essential to the onset and course of the illness. Preclinical and early clinical trials have yielded positive outcomes for several immunotherapies.

Using monoclonal antibodies, which are proteins made in laboratories that imitate the immune system's typical reaction to aberrant proteins, is one type of immunotherapy. By binding and selectively targeting amyloid-beta plaques, these antibodies aid in their removal from the brain and stop them from building up. Recent research has demonstrated that monoclonal antibodies, like gantenerumab and aducanumab, can slow down cognitive deterioration in people with early-stage Alzheimer's disease and lower levels of amyloid-beta plaque.

The administration of an amyloid-beta vaccine is an additional immunotherapy strategy. The goal of vaccines is to elicit an immune response directed against a particular target—in this case, amyloid-beta. Researchers seek to stop plaque development and slow down the progression of the disease by administering a vaccination that stimulates the immune system to identify and combat amyloid-beta. Although the amyloid-beta vaccination's clinical studies have demonstrated encouraging outcomes in terms of lowering amyloid-beta levels, more investigation is required to ascertain the vaccination's long-term efficacy and safety.

Gene treatments have emerged as a potential game-changer in the care of Alzheimer's disease, in addition to immunotherapies. Gene therapies include modifying or correcting defective genes that lead to the development of a disease by working with the patient's genetic material. Scientists have discovered a number of genes, including APP and ApoE4, that raise the chance of acquiring Alzheimer's. Researchers aim to lower the risk of Alzheimer's disease or slow down its progression by focusing on these genes.

Using viral vectors to transfer therapeutic genes to the brain is one method of gene therapy. Modified viruses known as viral vectors can successfully transfer genetic material to target cells while being safe for humans to handle. These treatments try to either add genes that improve the brain's capacity to remove aberrant proteins or replace damaged genes. Although Alzheimer's gene therapy is still in the preclinical stages, encouraging results from early experiments in animal models have raised optimism for further clinical trials.

Another area of study in the therapy of Alzheimer's disease is targeted medication therapies. The goal of these interventions is to create medications that specifically target the cellular processes and mechanisms involved in the aetiology of Alzheimer's disease. Solanezumab is one medication that targets the soluble form of amyloid-beta and works to stop the build-up of this protein in the brain. Even while solanezumab did not significantly improve outcomes in previous clinical trials, a reanalysis of the data indicated that those with milder types of the condition may benefit from it. To investigate its safety and effectiveness, more research is being done.

In addition to these particular treatments, scientists are investigating a variety of additional cutting-edge strategies. Using microbiome therapies to leverage the gut-brain connection, improving brain plasticity through cognitive training and stimulation, and disrupting amyloid-beta plaques with ultrasound are a few examples. These complementary and alternative therapies have the potential to improve the way Alzheimer's disease is managed overall and to improve the quality of life for those who have the illness.

Even though research on Alzheimer's disease is always changing, it's critical to view new treatments with cautious hope. Many of these therapies are still in the experimental phase, and before they can be deemed safe and effective treatments, they must undergo extensive testing and validation. Furthermore, because Alzheimer's disease is complex, management must be comprehensive and multimodal, involving lifestyle changes, psychosocial support, and holistic healthcare.

In conclusion, research into novel therapeutics and treatments that alter the course of disease offers hope in the battle against Alzheimer's. Early research on targeted medication interventions, gene therapies, and immunotherapies has produced encouraging findings. These treatments may eventually help those with Alzheimer's live longer by slowing the disease's progression. But it's important to keep in mind that these treatments are still in the experimental phase, and further investigation is required to ascertain their long-term safety and effectiveness. As the enigmas surrounding this intricate illness persist, I am resolute in advocating for a comprehensive strategy for managing Alzheimer's disease that includes lifestyle adjustments, self-care practises, and psychosocial support in addition to cutting edge treatments. By taking a holistic and integrative approach, we can enable Alzheimer's patients and their families to lead the best lives imaginable.

The Role of Artificial Intelligence in Alzheimer's Research

The core of AI's powers are machine learning algorithms. These algorithms don't require explicit programming; instead, they are made to learn from data and get better over time. Machine learning algorithms can be used in Alzheimer's research to sort through large datasets, including clinical, neuroimaging, and genetic data, to find hidden correlations and possible risk factors and biomarkers.

Early Alzheimer's disease identification and detection is one area in which AI has had a major impact. Early detection of Alzheimer's disease is essential to ensure prompt therapies that may slow down the illness's course. Artificial intelligence has demonstrated potential in detecting minute modifications to brain structure and function that take place in the preclinical phases of Alzheimer's disease, prior to the onset of symptoms. AI systems can assist medical professionals in making quicker and more accurate diagnoses, which improves illness management, by identifying these changes.

Another area where AI has shown to be extremely useful is data analysis. Massive volumes of data are produced by research on Alzheimer's disease from a variety of sources, such as genetics, brain imaging, and clinical evaluations. It might be difficult and time-consuming to manually analyse and interpret this data. Researchers will need to spend much less time and effort processing and analysing this data thanks to AI-powered data analysis tools. This makes it possible to conduct a more thorough and in-depth investigation, which could lead to the discovery of novel therapeutic targets and a greater knowledge of the illness.

Artificial Intelligence (AI) exhibits significant potential in forecasting the course and outcome of Alzheimer's patients. Artificial intelligence algorithms are able to recognise trends and variables that impact the course of a disease by examining longitudinal data from sizable patient cohorts. This helps medical practitioners to make more educated judgments about treatment and care by allowing them to more accurately forecast how a patient's condition may change over time. Additionally, AI can assist in identifying patients who may be more susceptible to specific problems, such as behavioural and psychological symptoms of dementia (BPSD), allowing for the improvement of their quality of life through early interventions.

Personalized medicine is one specific field where AI has the potential to have a big influence. Alzheimer's is a complicated and diverse illness, with individuals displaying a range of symptoms, rates of progression, and reactions to various therapies. AI systems are capable of analysing genetic data, lifestyle variables, and clinical data to create individualised treatment regimens for each patient. This not only improves patient outcomes and raises the likelihood of a successful course of therapy, but it also reduces the possibility of adverse consequences.

AI can also help in the creation of novel medications and treatments for Alzheimer's disease. Conventional methods for finding and developing new drugs are expensive and time-consuming, and many promising candidates don't prove to be highly effective in clinical trials. By finding novel target proteins or molecules that are related with the disease and forecasting the efficacy of potential treatment medicines, artificial intelligence (AI) helps expedite the drug discovery process. This has the potential to result in quicker and more efficient treatments for Alzheimer's patients by drastically reducing the time and money needed for drug development.

Although AI is certainly intriguing, it's important to remember that these technologies are intended to complement healthcare workers, not to replace them. AI algorithms are instruments that support decision-making, data analysis, and the development of individualised treatment plans. In order to give Alzheimer's patients comprehensive care, healthcare professionals' knowledge and human contact are still crucial.

In summary, it is impossible to overstate the importance of artificial intelligence in Alzheimer's disease research. Artificial Intelligence (AI) holds great promise to transform our comprehension and handling of diseases through data analysis, predictive modelling, and machine learning algorithms. AI provides enormous potential for enhancing patient outcomes and creating novel treatments, from early detection and diagnosis to forecasting disease development and customising therapy regimens. To provide the greatest care possible for Alzheimer's patients, it is crucial to move cautiously forward and make sure that new AI technologies are developed, verified, and incorporated into healthcare practises in an ethical manner.

Lifestyle Interventions and Prevention Strategies

Maintaining general wellbeing and lowering the risk of many diseases, including Alzheimer's disease, depend heavily on leading a healthy lifestyle. Getting enough sleep, controlling stress, avoiding dangerous substances, maintaining a balanced diet, and engaging in regular physical activity are all components of a healthy lifestyle. Regular physical activity has been demonstrated to enhance cognitive function and lower the risk of cognitive decline. Exercise improves memory and cognitive function, boosts blood flow to the brain, and encourages the development of new neurons. It is advised to perform 75 minutes of vigorous-intense aerobic activity or at least 150 minutes of moderate-intense aerobic activity each week. In order to enhance muscle strength and balance, strength training exercises are to be included at least twice a week. Engaging in a consistent fitness regimen can considerably lower a person's risk of Alzheimer's disease.

Maintaining brain health and lowering the risk of Alzheimer's Disease both benefit from a balanced diet. Promising effects have been observed in protecting cognitive function when the Mediterranean diet, which emphasises fruits, vegetables, whole grains, lean meats, and healthy fats, is followed. This diet is high in anti-inflammatory and antioxidant-rich foods that help lower inflammation and oxidative stress, two factors that are connected to Alzheimer's disease. Because fatty fish, such salmon, tuna, and sardines, are high in omega-3 fatty acids, eating fish has been linked to a decreased risk of Alzheimer's disease. Omega-3 fatty acids can enhance memory and cognitive function and are crucial for maintaining the health of the brain. Limiting processed foods, sugar-filled drinks, and saturated fats is also crucial because these items have been linked to an increased risk of cognitive impairment. People can fuel their brains and guard against Alzheimer's Disease by adopting a balanced diet.

Participating in cognitive activities is essential for maintaining brain health and preventing Alzheimer's disease, in addition to maintaining a healthy lifestyle. Building a reserve of cognitive talents through mental stimulation and cognitive engagement can act as a buffer against the consequences of neurodegeneration. Reading, solving puzzles, picking up new skills, learning to play an instrument, and interacting with others have all been linked to a lower risk of cognitive decline. These mental exercises stimulate the brain, encourage the development of new neural connections, and improve cognitive performance. Cognitive activities can be started at any time, and including them in daily routines can have a big impact on brain health.

In order to stop or postpone the start of Alzheimer's disease, risk reduction strategies must be put into place. Alzheimer's disease risk factors include obesity, diabetes, high cholesterol, and hypertension, among other chronic health issues. Reducing the risk of cognitive decline requires managing these disorders with medication, lifestyle changes, and routine check-ups. Furthermore, since the condition of the heart and blood vessels has a direct impact on brain function, it is imperative to evaluate and manage cardiovascular health. It is possible to considerably lower the risk of cognitive decline and Alzheimer's disease by maintaining healthy blood pressure, cholesterol, and blood sugar levels.

In addition to physical health, mental and emotional wellness are important factors in delaying Alzheimer's disease. Alzheimer's disease risk and cognitive impairment have been associated with long-term stress. It's critical to practise stress-reduction strategies including mindfulness, deep breathing, meditation, and relaxation-promoting hobbies. Getting support from close friends and family, going to counselling or therapy sessions, and taking care of oneself can all help people manage stress and lower their chance of developing Alzheimer's disease.

This section on lifestyle interventions and prevention tactics emphasises how crucial it is to manage Alzheimer's disease holistically. People can actively lower their risk of cognitive decline and Alzheimer's disease by adopting certain lifestyle modifications. A person can take charge of their health by committing to a lifestyle that supports general well-being and making educated decisions. People can protect their brain health and possibly delay or prevent the beginning of Alzheimer's Disease by combining risk reduction strategies, cognitive engagement, healthy lifestyle, and emotional well-being.

Ethical Considerations and Policy Implications

I have direct experience with the difficulties that Alzheimer's patients and their families have in my capacity as a physician and health and wellness coach. To give elderly people the greatest care possible, a number of ethical and policy-related concerns must be resolved in addition to the physical and cognitive deterioration.

Getting informed permission is one of the most crucial ethical factors in the treatment of Alzheimer's disease. It is unclear who should make decisions on behalf of Alzheimer's patients as they may eventually lose the capacity to make decisions regarding their own care. By giving their informed permission, patients may make sure they are aware of the advantages and disadvantages of their therapies as well as any other options that may be accessible to them. It enables people to keep their independence and make choices according with their preferences and values.

However, getting Alzheimer's patients' informed consent can be a difficult and delicate procedure. Patients may have trouble processing and remembering information as their illness worsens. It then becomes imperative to include family members or authorised healthcare proxies in the decision-making process in such circumstances. Simplified language and visual aids are two examples of communication tactics that might be useful in promoting understanding and getting informed consent.

Another crucial ethical factor in the treatment of Alzheimer's disease is privacy. As cognitive abilities deteriorate and dependence on others for daily tasks increases, people with Alzheimer's disease frequently suffer a loss of privacy. Healthcare professionals must strike a balance between patients' rights to privacy and dignity and the necessity to safeguard their safety and wellbeing. This could entail developing settings that encourage seclusion, including private rooms and personal areas in healthcare institutions. It also necessitates putting procedures in place to safeguard patients' private data and guaranteeing that only people with the proper authorization can access their medical records.

One important policy consideration in the treatment of Alzheimer's disease is access to care. As the number of cases of Alzheimer's disease rises, it is critical to make sure people can get the assistance and care they require. This covers not just medical care but also all-inclusive dementia care services like support groups, memory clinics, and respite care. Policies that cater to the special requirements of Alzheimer's patients and their families must be developed; they should include financial support services and programmes for caregivers. This will enhance the general standard of treatment and lessen the load on patients and their loved ones.

Entire dementia policies are required to handle the complex issues associated with Alzheimer's disease. These regulations ought to take social, economic, and legal factors into account in addition to the medical components of treatment. They ought to support early diagnosis and detection, foster innovation and research in Alzheimer's care, and offer standards for moral decision-making. Comprehensive dementia policy should also aim to reduce the stigma attached to Alzheimer's and develop a culture that is more accepting and helpful to those who are affected by the illness.

Taking into account the opinions and viewpoints of all parties concerned is essential for creating ethical and policy frameworks for managing Alzheimer's disease. Patients, relatives, medical professionals, researchers, legislators, and advocacy organisations are all included in this. We can create morally sound, patient-centered policies and practises by encouraging communication and cooperation across these disparate groups.

In conclusion, managing Alzheimer's disease critically depends on ethical issues and policy ramifications. People with Alzheimer's can get the best care and support by addressing concerns including informed consent, privacy, care access, and the requirement for thorough dementia policies. Healthcare professionals, legislators, and the general public must collaborate to establish a culture that recognises and upholds the rights and needs of people with Alzheimer's disease. We can only hope to meaningfully touch the lives of individuals impacted by this awful disease by taking an ethical and holistic approach.

Global Collaborations and Research Initiatives

I have had the honour of collaborating closely with numerous specialists from a variety of health and wellness domains in my capacity as a physician and health and wellness coach. My personal experience has taught me the value of teamwork and the strength of group efforts in the battle against Alzheimer's disease. My goal in this subchapter is to highlight the outstanding international partnerships and research projects that are opening doors to a better knowledge and treatment of Alzheimer's disease.

1. International Cooperation:

International collaboration is essential to the field of Alzheimer's Disease research in order to further scientific understanding and discover practical therapies. Due of the disease's complexity, international cooperation is required, with several nations contributing their distinct viewpoints, specialties, and resources. Cooperation amongst scientists, physicians, researchers, and politicians from other nations speeds up progress by facilitating the exchange of information, creative ideas, and data.

For example, the Global Alzheimer's Association Interactive Network (GAAIN) is a platform that facilitates data analysis and exchange about dementia across national and international borders. Through this effort, scientists can access and examine a sizable amount of data, which may reveal findings that would not otherwise be made in the context of solitary research efforts. Through the dismantling of geographical obstacles, GAAIN facilitates international cooperation and a group effort to discover practical treatments for Alzheimer's disease.

2. Data Sharing:

Data sharing is one of the most important aspects of international cooperation in Alzheimer's research. Making decisions in a subject that is always changing and where new discoveries are produced on a daily basis requires having access to extensive and current data. Researchers from different countries can share and pool resources through international collaborations, which helps them find trends and do more thorough studies than they could if they worked alone.

An excellent example of cooperative data sharing is the Alzheimer's Disease Neuroimaging Initiative (ADNI). The goal of this 2004 project was to facilitate the sharing of data obtained from neuroimaging, biomarkers, and clinical assessments among researchers in North America. Our knowledge of Alzheimer's disease has advanced thanks in large part to the shared data from ADNI, which has helped identify new therapy targets and enhanced diagnostic techniques.

In addition, the open access movement in science has gained strength and is now supporting the unrestricted dissemination of research results and data. Projects like PubMed Central and the Open Science Framework give researchers a platform to freely exchange their data, which promotes cooperation and study replication.

3. Collaborative Research Efforts:

Experts from a variety of professions collaborate in research projects to investigate various facets of Alzheimer's disease. Researchers can study the illness from a variety of perspectives by integrating their knowledge and experience, which can result in creative approaches to diagnosis, treatment, and prevention. These partnerships contribute to our understanding of the effects of genetics, environment, and lifestyle variables, as well as helping to unravel the fundamental processes of Alzheimer's disease.

The Dominantly Inherited Alzheimer Network is one prominent instance of cooperative research (DIAN). DIAN is a global research collaboration devoted to the study of people with dominantly inherited Alzheimer's disease (DIAN-AD), a rare type of the illness that develops earlier in life and is brought on by particular genetic abnormalities. The DIAN research community has made great progress in comprehending the early stages of Alzheimer's Disease, finding biomarkers, and investigating new therapeutic strategies by combining resources and exchanging data.

Furthermore, cooperation encompasses not only academic institutions but also governmental agencies, nonprofit groups, and pharmaceutical corporations. These collaborations support the creation of research networks, the advancement of clinical trials, and the practical implementation of discoveries. Through goal alignment, resource sharing, and harnessing individual skills, these collaborations produce a synergy that propels Alzheimer's research forward.

To sum up, international cooperation and research projects are essential to improving our knowledge of Alzheimer's disease and how to treat it. Scientists and medical professionals can transcend national borders, access a variety of viewpoints, and combine resources to advance their discipline through international cooperation, data exchange, and cooperative research projects. These programmes act as a ray of hope, showing us that by banding together, we can better tackle Alzheimer's Disease and enhance the lives of the millions of people who are afflicted by this terrible illness.

Hope for the Future: A World Without Alzheimer's

In an effort to comprehend the mechanics and causes of Alzheimer's disease, a great deal of study has been done throughout the years. These investigations have illuminated the role of lifestyle, environmental, and genetic factors in the development of this illness. With this understanding, we are better equipped to identify and diagnose Alzheimer's disease in its early stages, which is essential for efficient treatment and intervention.

Moreover, the progress made in the field of medicine has unlocked an extensive array of opportunities concerning prevention and therapy. Pharmaceutical companies and scientists are working nonstop to create medications that can either lessen the symptoms of the disease or halt its advancement. Even while there isn't a permanent solution yet, the current study provides us optimism that useful medicines will be developed soon.

Apart from pharmaceutical therapies, lifestyle adjustments have demonstrated their efficacy in the management and prevention of Alzheimer's disease. I have seen firsthand the life-changing effects of lifestyle modifications on individuals with Alzheimer's disease throughout my years of practise as a medical doctor and health and wellness consultant. Individuals can dramatically lower their risk of getting the condition or slow down its course by using a well-rounded approach that includes cognitive stimulation, regular exercise, healthy nutrition, stress reduction, and social involvement.

It is noteworthy that the joint endeavours of diverse healthcare practitioners have been crucial in the battle against Alzheimer's disease. We can guarantee that patients receive comprehensive care that takes into account all facets of their well-being by working with specialists from various health and wellness sectors. Experts such as dietitians, psychologists, counsellors, and practitioners of alternative medicine bring a variety of viewpoints and approaches to the table, which improves the overall standard of care provided to individuals with Alzheimer's disease.

It is imperative that we keep funding studies and clinical trials in the future to increase our comprehension of Alzheimer's disease. Through our financial support and active participation in clinical trials, we can help pave the way for the creation of ground-breaking therapies and interventions. Furthermore, promoting early detection, eradicating stigma, and motivating people to seek prompt medical assistance are all made possible by increasing public awareness of Alzheimer's disease.

Advocating for policies that prioritise Alzheimer's research, education, and support is equally crucial in our quest for a world free of Alzheimer's. Together, we can make a difference by speaking out and insisting that governments and healthcare institutions provide sufficient funding to address this urgent matter. It is imperative that all people impacted by Alzheimer's disease have access to reasonably priced care, specialist clinics, and support systems.

It is critical to stress the value of compassion and support for people with Alzheimer's disease and their families as we look forward to a time when this illness will no longer be a burden. Alzheimer's patients' loved ones are profoundly impacted by the disease in addition to the individual with the diagnosis. No one has to travel this path alone if we work to create a caring community that offers the required support networks.

To sum up, even if Alzheimer's disease can bring about a lot of difficulties, I really think that a world free of this illness is achievable. A better future may be possible if researchers, medical experts, legislators, and those impacted by Alzheimer's disease band together and work tirelessly. We can and will defeat Alzheimer's together if we band together in our fight against the illness, using hope as our driving force and working to build a society where everyone has access to effective prevention, treatment, and support.